THE CANCER WITHIN

MEDICAL ANTHROPOLOGY: HEALTH, INEQUALITY, AND SOCIAL JUSTICE

Series editor: Lenore Manderson

Books in the Medical Anthropology series are concerned with social patterns of and social responses to ill health, disease, and suffering, and how social exclusion and social justice shape health and healing outcomes. The series is designed to reflect the diversity of contemporary medical anthropological research and writing, and will offer scholars a forum to publish work that showcases the theoretical sophistication, methodological soundness, and ethnographic richness of the field.

Books in the series may include studies on the organization and movement of peoples, technologies, and treatments, how inequalities pattern access to these, and how individuals, communities, and states respond to various assaults on well-being, including from illness, disaster, and violence.

For a list of all the titles in the series, please see the last page of the book.

THE CANCER WITHIN

Reproduction, Cultural Transformation, and Health Care in Romania

CRISTINA A. POP

RUTGERS UNIVERSITY PRESS

New Brunswick, Camden, and Newark, New Jersey, and London

Library of Congress Cataloging-in-Publication Data

Names: Pop, Cristina Alexandra, 1973– author.
Title: The cancer within: reproduction, cultural transformation, and health
   care in Romania / Cristina A. Pop.
Other titles: Medical anthropology (New Brunswick, N.J.)
Description: New Brunswick: Rutgers University Press, [2022] | Series: Medical
   anthropology | Includes bibliographical references and index.
Identifiers: LCCN 2021038285 | ISBN 9781978829589 (paperback; alk. paper) |
   ISBN 9781978829596 (hardcover; alk. paper) | ISBN 9781978829602 (epub) |
   ISBN 9781978829619 (pdf)
Subjects: MESH: Uterine Cervical Neoplasms | Women's Health Services |
   Anthropology, Medical | Romania
Classification: LCC RC280.U8 | NLM WP 480 | DDC 616.99/466009498—dc23
LC record available at https://lccn.loc.gov/2021038285

A British Cataloging-in-Publication record for this book is available from the British
Library.

Figure 3 reprinted with permission, courtesy of Minerva Photographic Archives
of the Minerva Cultural Association, Cluj, Romania.

References to internet websites (URLs) were accurate at the time of writing. Neither
the author nor Rutgers University Press is responsible for URLs that may have expired
or changed since the manuscript was prepared.

♾ The paper used in this publication meets the requirements of the American National
Standard for Information Sciences—Permanence of Paper for Printed Library
Materials, ANSI Z39.48-1992.

www.rutgersuniversitypress.org

Manufactured in the United States of America

For Pavel and Letiția

CONTENTS

CONTENTS

FOREWORD

LENORE MANDERSON

Medical Anthropology: Health, Inequality, and Social Justice is concerned with the diversity of contemporary medical anthropological research and writing. The beauty of ethnography is its capacity, through storytelling, to make sense of suffering as a social experience and to set it in context. Central to our focus in this series, therefore, is the way in which social structures, political and economic systems, and ideologies shape the likelihood and impact of infections, injuries, bodily ruptures and disease, chronic conditions and disability, treatment and care, social repair, and death.

Health and illness are social facts; the circumstances of the maintenance and loss of health are always and everywhere shaped by structural, local, and global relations. Social formations and relations, culture, economy, and political organization as much as ecology shape the variance of illness, disability, and disadvantage. The authors of the books in this series are concerned centrally with health and illness, healing practices, and access to care, but in these different volumes, the authors highlight the importance of such differences in context as expressed and experienced at individual, household, and wider levels. Health risks and outcomes of social structure and household economy (for example, health systems factors), and national and global politics and economics, all shape people's lives. In their accounts of health, inequality, and social justice, the authors move across social circumstances, health conditions and geography, and their intersections and interactions to demonstrate how individuals, communities, and states manage assaults on people's health and well-being.

As medical anthropologists have long illustrated, the relationships of social context and health status are complex. In addressing these questions, the authors in this series showcase the theoretical sophistication, methodological rigor, and empirical richness of the field while expanding a map of illness, social interaction, and institutional life to illustrate the effects of material conditions and social meanings in troubling and surprising ways. The books reflect medical anthropology as a constantly changing field of scholarship, drawing on research diversely in residential and virtual communities, clinics and laboratories, and emergency care and public health settings, with service providers, individual healers, and households, and with social bodies, human bodies, biologies, and biographies. While medical anthropology once concentrated on systems of healing, particular diseases, and embodied experiences, today the field has expanded to include environmental disaster, war, science, technology, faith, gender-based violence, and forced migration. Curiosity about the body and its vicissitudes remains a pivot of our work, but our concerns are with the location of bodies in social life and with how social structures, temporal imperatives, and shifting exigencies shape life courses. This dynamic field reflects an ethics of the discipline to address these pressing issues of our time.

Globalization adds to the complexity of influences on health outcomes: It (re)produces social and economic relations that institutionalize poverty, unequal conditions of everyday life and work, and environments in which disease prevalence grows or subsides. It shapes health experiences and outcomes across space, informing and amplifying inequalities at individual and country levels. As Cristina Pop illustrates in *The Cancer Within*, globalization enables the transfer of technologies for cancer prevention and treatment. But the experiences of cancer, and access to these technologies, and the context in which cancer is understood—in this case, in relation to women's reproductive and sexual health—are no less determined by local histories, ideologies, and social relations.

As the subtitle of this series indicates, we are concerned with questions of social exclusion and inclusion, social justice and repair, again both globally and in local settings. The books will challenge readers not only to reflect on sickness and suffering, deficit and despair, but also on resistance and restitution—on how people respond to injustices and evade the fault lines that might seem to predetermine life outcomes. The aim is to widen the frame within which we conceptualize embodiment and suffering.

Romanian women are diagnosed with and die from cervical cancer consistently in higher and rising numbers compared to other women in Europe—at double the rates in countries with communist histories similar to Romania and far higher than in countries elsewhere in Europe. This book by Cristina Pop, *The Cancer Within: Reproduction, Cultural Transformation, and Health Care in Romania*, begins with this enigma.

Under the brutal communist regime of Nicolae Ceaușescu (1965–1989), even in the context of aggressive pronatalism (Kligman 1988), the state largely ignored women's reproductive health. With the overthrow of Ceaușescu in 1989, shifts to a free market economy, and Romania's entry into the European Union in 2007, the country's medical system transformed in ways that enabled both state and market services. Health care was consequently divided along predictable lines: public and private services, with quality of care and choice of provider tied to capacity to pay. In this context, Ceaușescu's legacy of the violent disregard of women undermined any ideological and institutional commitments to equality and justice. Patriarchal attitudes and state structures continued to shape policies concerned with women's health, including prenatal and postpartum care, childbirth, contraception, and abortion. Cervical cancer folded into this mix: It was seen as a stigmatizing pathology, with implications of sexual license. Hence, as before, under new forms of government policies and services, women's labor, sexuality, and reproductive bodies were scrutinized, subject to everyday forms of governance. Quality sexual and reproductive health care, and the fundamental values that shape their provision, continued into the twenty-first century to be deeply problematic. Cervical cancer's shocking metrics highlight this disparity of care.

While it is highly malignant, cervical cancer is a slow-growing cancer. Detection through Pap tests and human papillomavirus (HPV) screening allows for early diagnosis and successful treatment; the HPV vaccine allows for primary prevention. But because of its categorization as a sexually transmitted disease, cervical cancer is deeply stigmatized in Romania and elsewhere—both historically, when its etiology in human papillomavirus infection was not known, and subsequently, when it proved to be so. Attitudes to women of all ages valorize chastity, purity, and subjugation to men, resulting in the harsh judgment of those presumed to have flaunted codes of restrained behavior and leading to women's reluctance to present for screening or, in the face of signs of disease, to seek diagnosis, follow-up, treatment, and care. In addition, among poor communities, the exposure of purpose for women attending mobile units (described by Cristina Pop as she introduces us to her field site) discourages screening. Domestic circumstances and lack of temporal and financial resources to travel for health services, the challenges of intimate procedures, and for some women, the background memories of sexual abuse, further hinder decisions to seek care. Interventions such as colposcopy and cervical biopsy are not well understood (by most people), and the treatment pathways for cancer can be demanding.

The ethnographic field research against which Pop illustrates the complexities of care was conducted in the small town of Roșiorii de Vede, located to the southwest of Bucharest on the road to Bulgaria. Here, cancer's social life unfolds in the health system and its inequities at the community, family, and individual levels. Gender, poverty, and distrust unsettle women's confidence in health services, and they mute their health needs in the face of the cost of public exposure and the challenges of seeking care in a fraught, underfunded, and highly politicized system. Women experienced routine health services that left them embarrassed and sometimes humiliated. Pop's own experiences of obstetrics make clear the limits of reproductive and sexual health care even in metropolitan Romania.

The tragedy, as Pop illustrates for us, is that in the aftermath of communism, increasing inequalities in disseminating and accessing medical care have persisted, and these interact with other inequalities affecting women's life chances and their sexuality and reproductive health. Anthropologists have long attended to how illness, poor health outcomes, and early death track social fault lines, even if these tracks vary somewhat according to disease and country context. For women, inequalities in education, social and economic class, smoking, oral contraception use, and other factors combine and interact, loading onto each other, and recursively shape risk and influence speed of diagnosis and outcomes of disease (Manderson and Warren 2016). In Romania, these everyday vulnerabilities compound in cervical cancer. In describing this "perfect storm" of social and biological risks in this compelling and rich ethnography, Cristina Pop takes us to new ways to understand faith and economic precarity, fear, and unpredictability. *The Cancer Within* draws us into the ordinariness of everyday life and the echoes of a savage past, and the tragedies that play out in reproductive suffering and local gendered moralities.

NOTE ON TERMINOLOGY

Throughout this book, I follow historian Lucian Boia in using "communism" to refer to Romania's 1946–1989 political regime and "postcommunism" to designate the time period in the aftermath of 1989 until the present day. In doing so, I deviate from what has become the norm in anthropological studies written by western researchers who prefer to employ "socialism" and "post-socialism." As Boia shows (2016, 10), the term "communism" captures better the totalitarian nature of the Romanian government. The terminological distinction would also avoid confusions between Romania's political regime and versions of socialism found in some western European or Scandinavian countries.

THE CANCER WITHIN

INTRODUCTION
Systemic Contingencies

Midsummer, 2013. A white truck featuring an enormous pink ribbon sticker on its left side is traveling from the Romanian capital city of Bucharest to Roșiorii de Vede, in Teleorman County, on a three-day tour. Its journey has started in front of a massive red-brick concrete apartment building in downtown Bucharest—the headquarters of *Renașterea* ("The Rebirth"), a nongovernmental organization (NGO) that serves as a foundation for women's health.

The white truck is the foundation's mobile clinic. It provides women from rural and remote areas of Romania with free breast cancer and cervical cancer screenings. Among Romanian women between ages 15 and 44, breast cancer and cervical cancer are, respectively the first and second most common cancers and the leading causes of cancer deaths (Bruni et al. 2019). While Romania's breast cancer rates align with those of other European nations, cervical cancer statistics are exceptionally high. For several years, Romania experienced the highest cervical cancer incidence in the European Region, with a historic peak of 35.5 cases for every 100,000 women as recently as 2014, when the European average was 9.7 cases (table 1).

To put these numbers into perspective, Romania's 2014 cervical cancer incidence was triple the rates of the United Kingdom and Germany, and seven times higher than those of Finland, Italy, and Malta. A 2018 report places cervical cancer incidence in Romania at rates significantly higher than those of other eastern European countries such as Poland, Czechia, Russia, Ukraine, and Hungary (Bruni et al. 2019). The upswing in cervical cancer incidence in Romania contrasts with the overall decline of cases in the European Region. Furthermore, Romania's age-standardized mortality was consistently the highest of the European Region every year from 1972 to 2016. After reaching an all-time peak in 2002, with 15.4 deaths for every 100,000 women, compared to the European average of 4.6 deaths, mortality started to decline. Still, in 2014, out of every 100,000 Romanian women, 13 died of cervical cancer (table 2). These mortality rates are

TABLE 1.   Incidence of cervical cancer per 100,000.

	1994	1999	2000	2002	2003	2005	2008	2014
Romania	23.4	26.2	25	30.6	29.4	28.9	32.2	35.5
Southeastern Europe Health network members	19.1	20.9	20.6	23.2	22.7	22.1	24.6	24.9
WHO European Region	10.6	10.1	10.2	10.1	9.9	9.7	10.1	9.7

SOURCE: World Health Organization, European Health Information Gateway, https://gateway.euro .who.int/en/indicators/hfa_377-2360-incidence-of-cervix-uteri-cancer-per-100-000/visualizations /#id=19308.

TABLE 2.   Age-standardized deaths, cervical cancer per 100,000.

	1996	1998	2002	2003	2006	2007	2013	2014
Romania	14.6	14.9	15.4	15.2	14.7	14.5	12.9	13
Southeastern Europe Health network members	9.3	9.4	9.6	9.4	9.3	9.4	8.4	8.3
WHO European Region	4.9	4.8	4.6	4.5	4.3	4.4	4.2	4.2

SOURCE: World Health Organization, European Health Information Gateway, https://gateway .euro.who.int/en/indicators/hfa_144-1560-sdr-cancer-of-the-cervix-uteri-all-ages-per-100-000 /visualizations/#id=19073.

three times the European average and six times those of Spain, France, and Germany. Even compared to other eastern European countries, Romania's numbers are exceptional: almost three times higher than those of Czechia, double those of Hungary and Poland, and significantly higher than mortality rates recorded in neighboring countries such as Ukraine, Bulgaria, and Serbia (Apostol et al. 2010; Arbyn et al. 2010; Ilișiu et al. 2019; Bruni et al. 2019).

Cervical cancers cover a wide range of abnormal growth of the cell lining of the cervix—the lower part of the uterus. Most cervical cancers can either be similar to skin cancers or be produced by an abnormal proliferation of glandular tissue inside the cervix cells (American Cancer Society 2020). The main risk factor for developing cervical cancer is infection by the human papillomavirus (HPV), notably by HPV types 16 and 18, which are considered oncogenic because they can trigger the growth of malignant tumors. Most HPV infections, however, do not produce any abnormalities in the cervix structure. Cervical cancer is considered a slow-growing and silent type of cancer because the abnormal cells are unlikely to spread quickly to nearby tissue and often their growth does not produce any symptoms. Because cervical cancers tend to be asymptomatic, early detection—in the form of a Pap smear (Papanicolaou test) or HPV molecular screening—is crucial. When detected and treated at early stages—and sometimes even at later stages—cervical cancers have high rates of survival (Benard et al. 2017).

The truck slowly crosses the scorching asphalt of busy streets named after the nation's celebrated poets, until it reaches a wide boulevard, named for a famous general who fought the Ottomans. On the left, the truck passes the Bucharest National Theater, with the largest theater edifice in Europe, and the twenty-four-story Intercontinental Hotel. On the right, it passes the headquarters of the University of Bucharest. It turns and continues along another crowded boulevard, this one named after a German-born princess with a fondness for literature—the first queen of modern Romania. Upon crossing the river Dâmbovița, the truck follows a complicated path through the dusty maze of Bucharest streets, passing by huge concrete apartment buildings, neighborhood pizzerias, the giant glass cube of a luxury shopping mall, and a cemetery named after yet another nineteenth-century nationalist hero.

Romania's recent past, so noticeably evoked in the capital city's landmarks, has been marked by a series of major historical changes. After its provinces gained independence from the Ottoman Empire at the end of the nineteenth century and from the Austro-Hungarian Empire in the aftermath of World War I, Romania became a constitutional monarchy, ruled by naturalized kings from the German House of Hohenzollern who converted to Eastern Orthodoxy (figure 1).

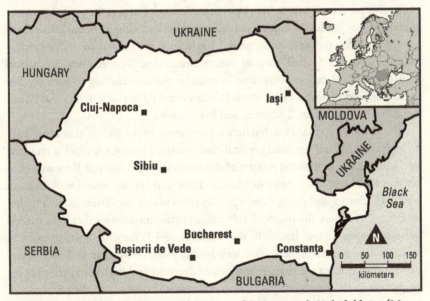

FIGURE 1. Map of Romania showing the location of the Roşiorii de Vede field site. (Map by Eureka Cartography.)

After World War II, a Soviet-backed government overturned the monarchy and instituted a communist regime that lasted for over four decades. In 1965, communist dictator Nicolae Ceaușescu came to power. He ruled the country in a totalitarian style until December 1989, when he was ousted from power and executed during a violent anti-communist mass revolt. Following a difficult postcommunist transition, Romania joined the European Union (EU) in 2007. These historical transformations have left enduring legacies that extend well beyond urban geographies; they permeate everyday practices that shape ordinary people's lives, health, and well-being.

In accounting for Romania's cervical cancer statistics, epidemiologists point to the likely role of historical transformations in placing particular generations of women at high risk. These include changes in sexual behavior, enhanced by smoking and/or oral contraception use (Arbyn et al. 2010). Women born in eastern Europe and central Asia between 1940 and 1960 share similar and generation-specific cervical cancer mortality trends (Ginsburg et al. 2017; Bray et al. 2005). Romania appears to be part of a geographical area with a demonstrated endemic prevalence of the HPV oncogenic genotype 16 (De Sanjosé et al. 2007; Ilișiu et al. 2019). Other scholars note that the recent historical transformations have increased the cervical cancer burden in eastern Europe by creating unequal access to screening, as part of the postcommunist reforming of health care (Todorova et al. 2006). As Andreassen and her collaborators (2017) demonstrate in a study among Romanian Roma, in some cases, the local mismanagement of cervical cancer screening inadvertently reproduces ethnic stigma, leading women to decline from participating in free preventive exams. As elsewhere in eastern Europe, the postcommunist transition has produced unprecedented social and economic inequalities. These emergent socioeconomic and cultural landscapes are critical to understanding people's attitudes toward cervical cancer prevention. For instance, Romanian women's cervical cancer prevention knowledge varies according to their level of education and socioeconomic status (Crăciun and Băban 2012; Pența and Băban 2013; Pop 2016; Crăciun, Todorova, and Băban 2018).

The scholarship that I quoted here reveals some of the factors that contribute to high regional and national cervical cancer rates. However, we lack a nuanced and historically articulated picture of the reasons that single out Romania even among its closest European neighbors. How can we account for Romanian women suffering and dying from a mostly preventable condition in such higher numbers? What are the political, cultural, and structural forces that have shaped women's reproductive health in the last decades? Where are men situated in relation to women's reproductive well-being? How do secular and nonsecular rationalities inform women's reproductive decision-making? What are people's responses to the emergent postcommunist transformations in the provision of both public and private reproductive care? Why are Romanians constantly glossing over the moralities of reproduction and reproductive care?

Anthropologists increasingly consider cancer through a biocultural lens, challenging generic descriptions of oncologic medicine. A plurality of "anthropologies of cancer" (Mathews, Burke, and Kampriani 2015) can better account for the fact that living with cancer amounts to intimate experiences both "within and outside of the body" (Manderson 2015, 247).

Culturally and historically situated, the lived experiences of cancer "as something that happens *between* people" (Livingston 2012, 6) are fundamentally intersubjective. Cancer seizes the collective imagination (Jain 2013) and people establish connections between cancer and the natural environment, kinship networks, and the moral value of life. For instance, to the farmers in a southwest Chinese village, "the fight against cancer . . . is deeply bound to efforts not only to maintain health but also to debate one's position within the family and the local community" (Lora-Wainwright 2013:6). In the United States and elsewhere, as individuals reimagine their postsurgical bodies following cancer interventions (Manderson 1999, 2011), survivorship emerges as a form of identity around the idea that "cancer becomes us" (Jain 2013). While cancer etiologies are historical, they are not immutable (Lora-Wainwright 2013). Cancer patients may actively imagine emergent forms of biosociality, the way thyroid cancer survivors did in post–Chernobyl Ukraine, when they reconsidered ideas about personhood and belonging in relation to suffering (Petryna 2003). Furthermore, a cancer diagnosis may drive patients to reconsider the value of biomedicine itself (Chavez et al. 1995; Lende and Lachiondo 2009) and to examine "who claims knowledge about cancer and how" (Jain 2013, 5).

Ethnographies of cancer scrutinize the available technologies of prevention, diagnosis, and treatment. As the focus shifts away from conceptualizing cancers in epidemiological terms—such as being "at risk"—cancers are progressively seen through the lens of embodied structural vulnerability (Armin, Burke, and Eichelberger 2019). Living with cancer illuminates the broad inequalities in the provision of health care that affect structurally vulnerable populations such as uninsured and/or undocumented patients in the United States (Armin 2015, 2019). This approach also challenges ethnocentric assumptions about oncologic medicine and highlights the political and moral economy embedded in the provision of health care. The precarious infrastructure of the only cancer ward in Botswana exposes biomedicine as "an incomplete solution" and improvisation as the main feature of oncology in low-income countries (Livingston 2012). In rural northeast Thailand, the communication of a cancer diagnosis and the management of palliative care observe localized bioethics discourses that surround dying of cancer (Bennett 1999; Boonmongkon, Pylypa, and Nichter 1999). These anthropologies of cancer reveal the uneven global distribution of biomedical technologies, as well as the multiplicity of ways in which authoritative knowledge about cancer and its prevention and cure gets translated into practice.

Anthropological interest in cervical cancers is shaped in specific ways by cultural meanings attached to the particular anatomy of the cervix and the oncological specificity of cervical cancers when compared to other types of cancers (Wood, Jewkes, and Abrahams 1997; Martinez, Chavez, and Hubbell 1997; Chavez et al. 2001; Gregg 2011). Cervical cancers (and perhaps all gynecological cancers) are intimately tied to reproductive health. Cervical cancer's connection to reproductive health fleshes out the central argument of this book—that Romanians' resistance to cervical cancer prevention is situated not so much in relation to cancer itself but to the historical and personal unfolding of their reproductive lives. The cervix is a liminal reproductive organ through which bodily fluids either flow from the uterus to the vagina (menstrual blood) or are directed from the vagina to the uterus (sperm). Hidden in a woman's body, the cervix is one of those organs that is typically surrounded by "a deep cultural horror of what is inside, a terror of female genitals and the space behind them" (Kapsalis 1997,126). Because the cervix is invisible even to women themselves, "the politics of seeing the cervix" is deeply medicalized and it stages an asymmetric power relation between women and their doctors—as only the latter perform the cervical display (Kapsalis 1997).

While the cervix is invisible to women, cervical cancer is often described as a silently growing cancer. Yet, unlike the other silent killers such as lung, ovarian, and colorectal cancer, cervical cancer can be detected at early stages through the Pap smear, a cost-effective and simple routine procedure. However, in the absence of symptoms, some women may perceive the Pap smear an unnecessary biomedicalization of their sexual and reproductive bodies rather than a procedure to their benefit. For instance, in Brazilian favelas, women challenge the very notion of medical risk related to cervical cancer as long as not being at risk for cervical cancer allows them to tactically use sex to acquire desired security and freedom (Gregg 2003).

Cervical cancer is one of the very few cancers linked to an identifiable viral pathogen, the human papillomavirus. Infection with HPV is the most common sexually transmitted infection (STI) worldwide. Since, in some cases, HPV will cause cervical cancer, there is a strong connection between cervical cancer and STIs. This link often reinforces stigmatizing narratives about this type of cancer, even among medical experts. Such is the case among Bulgarian and Romanian medical practitioners whose moralizing discourses around women's (lack of) participation in cervical cancer prevention revolve around allegations of sexual promiscuity (Todorova et al. 2006). Similarly, in Venezuelan doctors' and patients' cervical cancer risk profiling narratives, morality unevenly infuses discourses about sexuality, hygiene, and poverty. While patients emphasize the effects of economic inequalities on their access to cervical cancer early detection, doctors privilege stigmatizing discourses about loose sexuality and lack of sanitation (Martinez 2018).

In many parts of the world, Romania included, the politics of cervical cancer prevention has been informed by a neoliberal agenda of medical care reforms designed to cut health care costs by focusing on prevention and primary care. The neoliberal restructuring of the early detection of cervical cancer across Latin America, and especially in 1990s Venezuela, has prompted women to redefine agency and to resist testing (Martinez 2018). Worldwide, resistance to cervical cancer prevention intensified after primary prevention was developed in 2006 in the form of an HPV vaccine (Wailoo et al. 2010). The vaccine became immediately controversial at a global scale. Some of the parents of the prepubescent girls targeted by the vaccine distribution contested the notion that their daughters might have been at risk for cervical cancer. They also challenged pharmaceutical companies' claims that the HPV vaccine would prevent cervical cancer (Towghi 2013; Gottlieb 2018).

> The truck soon reaches the outskirts of the city where warehouses, parking lots, car dealership showrooms and franchise gas stations alternate with strips of landfill. The occasional pack of stray dogs can be seen in a brand-new suburb of salmon-painted villas, wandering along mud-covered side streets. After passing a tiny ABC supermarket, a shady nightclub, and a cheap bed-and-breakfast, the truck crosses a railway and picks up speed as it heads toward the southwest, along the European route E70, through a vast and flat landscape—the Bărăgan Plain.

As elsewhere in eastern Europe, recent historical changes are particularly visible in Romania's hybrid peri-urban zones. Here, emergent networks of upward and downward mobility have produced chaotic and fragmented landscapes where the global and the local often coexist. Ethnographers of postcommunism describe Bucharest's margins as spaces of boredom, homelessness, fast-food consumption, and shopping mall consumerism (O'Neill 2017).

I build my own ethnography of the changing landscapes of reproductive health care in contemporary Romania on such scholarship of postcommunist transformations, as well as on medical anthropology and public health literature. I look at cervical cancer prevention as a paradoxical locus not only for intersection but also disconnection between local and global discourses and practices. The Romanian cervical cancer case is a point of entry into a productive anthropological reflection on contemporary health care delivery. More than straightforward biomedical measures, cervical cancer screening and HPV vaccination reveal the inner workings of an emerging medical system that aligns the state and the market, public and private health care providers, policy makers, and ordinary women.

Throughout this book I denaturalize the fact that the lived experiences of being vaccinated against HPV, of being screened for abnormal cervical cell growths, or of suffering from cervical cancer have often been construed as contradictions. Such contradictions opposed long-term invisibility to early detection, sexuality to reproduction, STI to cancer, and patriarchal stigma surrounding a disease thought to be linked to promiscuous behavior to compassion for a pathology affecting a life-bearing body part. I integrate findings from ethnography and recent history to expand—rather than simplify in binary oppositions—the dimensions of human experience that are critical to our understanding of social processes, including disease.

I make three contributions to the conundrum of the cervical cancer burden in Romanian women. First, I go beyond narrow perspectives that label cervical cancer statistics as either "endemic" or "epidemic," and I complicate previous explanations of the burden of this disease among Romanian women. I argue that Romania's remarkably high cervical cancer incidence and mortality rates are the product of a series of social, historical, and health "co-occurrences" that point to syndemic circumstances. A concept first advanced by medical anthropologist Merrill Singer in 1994, a syndemic integrates social, political, and economic forces into an "explanatory model" (Good 1994) that challenges biomedical and public health approaches to disease as a discrete biological entity. In this understanding, social and biological factors reinforce each other through "mutually enhancing" interactions (Singer 1994). Unlike endemic or epidemic approaches, which are unidimensional, a syndemic is "a confluence of multiple health and social issues that interact to result in disproportionate rates of disease in vulnerable populations" (Kelly, Allison, and Ramaswamy 2018, 8). Similarly, to account for mutual conditionings between poverty, social exclusion and multiple chronic conditions, Manderson and Warren (2016) propose the concept of "recursive cascade." A term borrowed from information technology, a recursive cascade captures the dynamic that allows new health and social variables to continuously impact and reshape one's (pre)existing health and social conditions (Manderson and Warren 2016, 491). The type of phenomena encapsulated in the notions of "syndemic" and "recursive cascade" would be best approximated in lay terms by the metaphor of the "perfect storm."

In the case of cervical cancer in Romania, the "synergistic interaction[s] of diseases and social conditions" (Singer and Clair 2003, 423) are produced by what I call "systemic contingencies."[1] The idea of systemic contingencies partly overlaps with syndemic (and its focus on the impact of structural forces on one's health), recursive cascade (with its complicated interweaving of social and health trajectories), and perfect storm (with its inescapable alignment of variables). However, in proposing "systemic contingencies" as a distinct concept, I recognize that, beyond structural forces and trajectories, significant accidents take place, and these accidents are nevertheless historical, not "natural." Most of the instances I examine in *The Cancer Within* are systemic. They reflect the workings of structural forces whose manifestations have unfolded historically—such as official reproductive policies (chapter 1), patriarchal practices and attitudes regarding women's sexuality and reproduction (chapter 2), secular and nonsecular understandings of risk and prevention (chapter 3), medical care reforms (chapters 4 and 5), and allegations and suspicions of corruption (chapter 6). Although systemic, these forces are contingent: They make visible the unpredictability and ordinariness of everyday life. Let me enumerate just a few of the "facts of life" that women shared with me. To elude reproductive surveillance, Oana keeps both a real and a false record of her last menstruation (chapter 1). Ileana's husband and her in-laws confiscate the festive dishes that she prepared for a religious holiday and exclude her from the feast (chapter 2). On a closer X-ray examination, the suspected TB mark on one of Maria's lungs turns out to be the scar of a rib broken years ago during an episode of domestic violence (chapter 2). After giving birth to a premature baby, Ana fakes an attack of hysteria in order to be released early from the public maternity hospital (chapter 4). When the neonatal intensive care unit of a Bucharest hospital is left unattended, a devastating fire severely burns eleven premature newborns (chapter 6). Xenia's daughter travels abroad to earn the remittances for the bribery that a gynecologist had requested for Xenia's cancer surgery (chapter 6). How do these and similar stories of everyday life make sense, without acknowledging that they both reveal and obscure broader power relations? More importantly, in what ways do the systemic contingencies articulated through these stories inform our understanding of cervical cancer in Romania?

Second, I locate Romania's cervical cancer problem not in the field of oncogenesis and oncologic care but in the realm of reproduction and its moralities. A central part of my argument is that unparalleled traumatic state intervention into women's reproductive lives has shaped the way that women deal with their bodies and health and the ways that they engage with the medical system. I am concerned not so much with the quantifiable causes of cervical cancer incidence and mortality, as with cancer's "conditions of possibility" (Kant [1781] 2018), which are rendered (or not) apparent, over time, through social and cultural transformation. In my effort to capture the latent spectrality of recent history unfolding, I employ "hauntology" (Derrida [1994] 2006) as "a language for exploring ways of simultaneously knowing and not knowing, of the politics, suppressions, and ghostly appearances of contested memory" (Good 2020, 419). Romanian women's encounters with cervical cancer prevention often take place around institutions that resemble the "palimpsestic structures with prior lives and histories of violence" described elsewhere (Varley and Varma 2018:631). Drawing on Foucault's genealogic understanding of history as a means of engagement with the present, I examine cervical cancer in Romania as the embodiment of a veiled rationality from the recent past that "emerged out of specific struggles, conflicts, alliances, and exercises of power" (Garland 2014, 372). On a fundamental level, this is a book about emergence (Foucault 1977), a concept that I capture in the notion of the cancer *within*.

Third, like other medical anthropologists, I strive to convey a nuanced understanding of what suffering entails. Unlike some of my peers, however, I do not often find myself in a position to challenge sensationalistic media accounts. Some anthropologists demystify philanthrocapitalist representations of "superlative sufferers" (Heller 2019), and in doing so, they produce more complicated pictures of their research participants' lives, de-emphasizing desolation and abuse (Block and McGrath 2019). As citizens of a EU nation-state, Romanian women at risk of developing cervical cancer are not well suited to mediatic othering. Their bodies do not bear any visible, terrifying signs of a condition that may be unknown even to themselves. They are "ordinary sufferers," unsuitable as poster images of affliction. My endeavor involves recognizing how these unspectacular forms of reproductive vulnerability contribute to illuminating localized perceptions of global practices, meaningful resistance to enforced procedures, emergent social dynamics, and ultimately Romania's cervical cancer crisis. As we shall see, the women featured in this book are anything but ordinary.

Lowland villages fly by, with their slate-roofed houses, tidy vegetable gardens, and wide sunflower fields. Here and there, small Orthodox churches punctuate the landscape with their golden onion cupolas. On the narrow road shoulder of E70, women wheel carts packed with refilled propane tanks for their stoves. Children chase noisy geese, while donkeys graze on dusty, withered grass. Seated in plastic chairs in front of the "universal store," men savor cheap beer. Teenagers lounge near the local postal office. From the fast-moving truck, one can see multicolor plastic strips dangle at the open doors of bars and stores to keep out flies.

I grew up in a large and relatively cosmopolitan urban area of northern Romania, but I find the journey of the Renașterea truck through the rural southern plains deeply nostalgic. Although the 1980s were for most Romanians a time of extreme economic hardship and political oppression, my parents did their best to take my brother and me on countless road trips throughout the country. With a portable gas stove and dozens of cans of SPAM stored in its trunk, our overheated Dacia—the one and only national car brand—slowly crept through a landscape of fields and villages not unlike the one that the white truck drove through decades later.

As a native doing "fieldwork without malaria pills" (Hannerz 2006, 24), I struggled constantly to acknowledge and alter my bias (Iosif 2003; Mishtal 2015). Although differently situated, I am one of the Romanian women whose experiences with sexual and reproductive medicine I recount in this book. For this reason, in chapters 4, 5, and 6, I include excerpts from my own recollections of navigating the often-confusing landscapes of medical care in my native country. These "confessional tales" are woven here and there into the book, as a counterpoint to both the "realist tales" told by official public health statistics and the "impressionist tales" that women shared with me (Van Maanen 2011). My voice, of someone born in a province shaped by an Austro-Hungarian historical legacy, brings a rather dissonant note to the chorus of southern, peri-urban women from Roşiorii de Vede, who live in the county of Teleorman, once occupied by the Ottomans. Together, our stories speak of plural yet similar experiences; we challenge monolithic and essentializing accounts of the postcommunist "transition to democracy."

My personal experiences of sexual and reproductive medicine are typical for many women of my generation. Growing up under a communist regime, I learned that the official claims about women's health and well-being were mostly propaganda. One of my most poignant memories of the years when the dictator Ceauşescu led the country is the moment of my first menstruation. In the late 1980s, planned power outages were routine in the evenings. So it happened that one night, shivering with cold, then fright and emotion, in the darkness of the bathroom, I discovered menarche spots on my underwear. I called my mother to assist me. There was a shortage of cotton, and nobody had heard of absorbent pads. In the dim light of a couple of thin beeswax candles that she placed on the edge of the bathtub, my mother improvised a cloth from some old, shredded bed sheets. I watched her gentle folding movements. She handed me the cloth, whispering with bitter irony, more to herself than to me: "The [Communist] Party cares for women's well-being." Her words unintentionally marked my rite of passage to womanhood—a dreaded condition, as I would gradually realize.

As a teenager suffering from dysmenorrhea (that is, painful menstruation), I ended up several times in the emergency room of one of the local gynecological hospitals of Cluj-Napoca, a large university city of about 400,000. Because these consultations took place both before and after 1989, over time I was subjected to medical procedures that reflected first the reproductive policies of the communist rule and then, with the regime's fall, a sudden shift in sexual and reproductive care. Until December 1989, every time I went to the hospital, usually late at night, I had to wait for my turn. My body contorted with pain, I sat next to a freezing cold radiator, under the flicker of a defective fluorescent light, in an emergency room with chipped painted walls. The doctor, always a male gynecologist, always wrapped in a thick wool robe on top of his gown, would eventually give me analgesics through an IV and send me home, not before reminding me that my condition would improve once I gave birth. Given the unofficial but effective ban on modern contraception under Ceauşescu's pronatalist regime between 1967 and 1989, the only long-term treatment envisioned by the doctor for my painful menstruation was the hormonal changes that naturally occur during pregnancy and birth.

In May 1990, just months after the end of the pronatalist policies and the liberalization of abortion and modern contraception, my mother took me to one of the newly founded obstetrics and gynecology private practices in the city. The consultation room was nested in a tiny apartment of an eight-floor apartment building. A cheerful male OB-GYN gave me (and my mother) a ten-minute crash course in sex education and prescribed me contraceptive pills. In the following years, I was a patient of the newly created NGO Society for Contraceptive and Sexual Education (*Societatea de Educație Contraceptivă și Sexuală*, or SECS). SECS offered subsidized gynecological consultations and contraception. Every three months, to get my contraceptive pills supply renewed at discounted prices, I would take the trolley to a working-class residential neighborhood on the outskirts of the city. The discreet sign at the entrance of a dilapidated concrete apartment building—of a cartoonish face with female and male gender symbols as cheeks—made me feel like I was engaging in an illicit activity. Later, I started attending a private practice for my annual medical examination. Its owner, a male OB-GYN of rising professional status, had recruited me during one of my emergency visits in the public hospital, where he was also appointed full-time. More recently, while doing fieldwork in Roșiorii de Vede, I had an emergency pregnancy check-up in the local public hospital in September 2006, as I recount in chapter 6, and a consultation in the only OB-GYN private practice of the town, in October 2009. My reproductive health experiences also include several episodes of hospitalization, from a few hours to a week, in a state maternity hospital of Cluj-Napoca. Between 2002 and 2009, I was admitted for a miscarriage, a myomectomy (that is, a surgical procedure to remove uterine fibroids), a suspected miscarriage, four episodes of suspected preterm labor, and two C-section deliveries. After my second delivery, I had a routine check-up in a private maternity hospital in Cluj-Napoca. My endeavor of recalling some of these experiences in chapters 4 and 5 is facilitated and rendered more accurate by the field notes I took at the time of these various medical episodes.

As the truck approaches its destination, two identical silhouettes of furnaces from the bankrupt ROBEMA beer factory appear in the distance. The dilapidated furnaces—known to locals as "the twin towers," in a typical example of macabre humor—watch over the now ghostly factory. Upon entering Roșiorii de Vede, the truck passes by a deserted field where a group of traveling Roma has set up their temporary camp. A few women and kids sit by a smoky hearth. Wet laundry flutters on a rope attached to their wagons. Two scrawny horses of a dirty shade of white graze nearby.

During the early stages of my fieldwork, with Romania joining the EU in 2007 and the postcommunist transition presumably coming to an end, I thought that, in some ways, I was doing "salvage ethnography." I was probably witnessing the last sightings of itinerant Roma before their wagons were banned from European roads and the last images of industrial ruins before they were torn down in the name of EU-funded development. At that time, I was fascinated with the classic twentieth-century anthropology that produced systematic ethnological research of distinct communities (Bennett 1998). I imagined myself mapping women's sexual and reproductive health knowledge and practice in a small peri-urban community that I had a priori postulated as contained and self-sufficient. As often happens in empirical research, "accident and happenstance shape field-workers' studies as much as planning or foresight" (Van Maanen 2011, 2). During the summer of 2009, several women I was interviewing brought up the HPV vaccine in our conversations, attempting to elicit my opinion about a controversial national vaccination campaign that the government had launched the previous year. I am neither the first nor the last anthropologist to find herself interviewed by her research subjects, but upon hearing these women talking unprompted about an issue that concerned them, I realized that I had found the real point of entry into my research. Inquiring about the local responses to the HPV vaccine would soon lead me to discover the various transnational connections that linked this small peri-urban community of southern Romania to global discourses and practices.

While doing fieldwork, I was forced to reconsider the very notion of "place"[2] as the locus of my research. To better gauge the way women used virtual resources, such as online doctor reviews or hospital preparation advice, I accompanied them in "non-places" (Augé 2009) such as the internet. Such inquiries de-territorialized my research to a certain extent. Also, some of these women were only intermittently present in certain locations and were otherwise engaged in various trajectories of mobility. Oana, who I introduce in chapter 1, moved back and forth between Italy and Romania before finally settling back in Roşiorii de Vede after renovating her house with the euros she had earned abroad. Ileana, featured in chapter 2, confessed to me that her household was very much dependent on the money and goods that her two sons were sending periodically from Bucharest. Similarly, Maria, a key study participant who I discuss especially in chapters 2 and 3, received monthly remittances from her sons in Spain. Xenia's relatives, featured in the gossip that I reproduce in chapter 6, would partake in transnational economic migration to secure the informal payments supposedly granting her adequate medical care in Roşiorii de Vede hospital. Despite people being partly absent, places were increasingly saturated with the presence of other places (Mihăilescu 2007). Some of the actual health care delivery spaces that I observed in Roşiorii de Vede and elsewhere were in fact interconnected to other distant places, as a result of administrative attempts to comply with the "European standards" of care and to participate in an emergent consumerist culture of providing "medical services." However, the would-be presence of clean, well-endowed, and functional western clinics is complicated and sporadic in most public Romanian hospitals, as I suggest in the account of the sanitary inspection in Roşiorii de Vede OB-GYN hospital section from chapter 6 and in the other two personal vignettes in chapters 4 and 5.

Conducting anthropological fieldwork that involved discussing biomedical procedures and their alleged health benefits placed me in an ambiguous ethical position (Dilger, Huschke, and Mattes 2015). I am not a medical expert, but I am the mother of a daughter who one day may well receive the HPV vaccination. At times, I struggled to navigate between neither openly endorsing nor rejecting procedures like the Pap smear and the HPV vaccination. As with other ethnographers who study cervical cancer prevention, I aim to ultimately contribute to the literature that acknowledges the complicated, uneven responses to the intended health benefits of vaccination and screening (see also Todorova et al. 2006). Some women were rather evasive in our conversations, as they may have suspected me of pushing on them a cervical cancer prevention agenda. Occasionally, they elicited from me "the correct answer" to my own questions to them. A few challenged me to express my personal views on the HPV vaccination. In some cases, women would ask me questions in ways that I understood to be quite sarcastic. Such was the case when seventy-four-year-old Maria asked me whether I was afraid that I would get fined if I refused the HPV vaccine for my daughter. The question was ironic, since it implied that, unlike in the communist past, such a repressive scenario would be an absurdity in the present. Maria's sarcasm provided me with an insight into her views on past and present power relations between state authority and ordinary women. Her question encapsulated an implicit critique of a weakened postcommunist state, unable to manage the well-being of its young citizens.

> The truck creeps slowly along cracked and dusty streets, past a cemetery, bucolic houses with bountiful gardens, and concrete apartment buildings whose sealed balconies look like miniature space capsules, until it finally reaches its destination—the downtown area of Roșiorii de Vede, a town of 30,000 residents in Teleorman County.

This book is based on research conducted between 2005 and 2013 during several fieldwork seasons in Delcel (pronounced del-čel), a neighborhood of Roșiorii de Vede. A large rural locality of a certain commercial and geostrategic significance for most of its medieval and modern history, Roșiorii de Vede—also spelled Roșiori de Vede, and known simply as Roșiori—is situated about eighty miles southwest of Bucharest. Roșiorii de Vede underwent a process of accelerated industrialization in the 1960s and 1970s and was promoted to a higher administrative and economic ranking in 1995, through recognition as a "municipality" (*municipiu*). Like other small towns forcibly urbanized under communism, Roșiorii de Vede has experienced a halted development and even re-ruralization in the last three decades. After dismantling the town's heavy industries post-1989, unemployment soared among the working class, producing rippling effects among other socioeconomic groups, as professionals such as doctors, teachers, and engi-

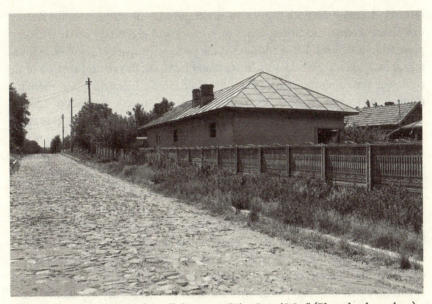

FIGURE 2. Street in Delcel informally known as "The Goats' Way." (Photo by the author.)

neers started to commute to Bucharest. From the early 2000s and especially since 2007, when Romania became part of the EU, many Roșioreni have engaged in transnational seasonal or more permanent migration to western European countries. Today, a significant percentage of the population practices subsistence agriculture in small gardens or on larger lots in neighboring villages.

The district of Delcel, situated in the southern periphery of Roșiorii de Vede and crossed by the Bratcov River—a muddy, meandering water stream— consists of about 200 households. Its residents, mostly working class of recent rural descent, include a majority of ethnic Romanians and a minority of Roma. Delcel was connected to electricity in the late 1960s and to natural gas in 2006. Despite these transformations, wood stoves remain the main heating source during typically harsh winters. As recently as 2012, Delcel did not have a sewage system or access to clean running water (figure 2). At the time of my fieldwork, few Delcel families had indoor bathrooms and most used pit latrines.

On a light traffic day, it takes about two hours to cover the eighty miles between Bucharest and Roșiorii de Vede. However, as the Renașterea mobile clinic was traveling to provide preventive sexual and reproductive care, time unfolded gradually, spanning over decades of momentous changes. During the trip from Bucharest to Roșiorii de Vede, the mobile-clinic-turned-time-machine traveled back to Romania's recent past.

When I started this study, I aimed to scrutinize Romania's puzzling high rates of cervical cancer incidence and mortality, seen as epidemiological problems apt to be explained from a biocultural and historical perspective. As part of my research, I examined both the macro-structural and the micro-political factors that shape women's local responses to primary and secondary cervical cancer prevention programs. I also considered the potential impact of small-scale findings at national and global levels. This inquiry lent itself to a critical analysis of an emergent postcommunist medical culture of claims, belonging, and mobility through the lens of market-shaped yet state-granted "health citizenship" (Porter 2011). When considered from the perspective of Romania's cervical cancer prevention programs, health citizenship reveals how the intricate dynamic of rights and responsibilities shapes not only ordinary people's practices in seeking health care but also their understandings of the changing moral landscapes of medicine.

As my research progressed, culturally situated temporalities became an overarching theme. What keeps together the multiple threads that I examine in the following pages are the past traumas that haunt the present time to the extent of hindering Romanians' attempts at imagining and pursuing a better future. As others have before me, I explore not only "the pastness of the past but its presence" as well (Eliot [1921] 1997, 28; see also Fassin 2007). The presumed linearity of chronological time is replaced with a traumatic lived history experienced as a constellation of entangled events. The people who populate *The Cancer Within* are children born to fulfill a destiny that an official state decree had already planned on their behalf; young women so overburdened with the restrictions of their reproductive rights that they express the wish to age prematurely; men who exert patriarchal prerogatives without taking responsibility for the reproductive consequences of their own sexuality; newborns burned to death in a maternity hospital; ordinary citizens who anchor their anxieties over imagined food contamination in past environmental disasters; and mothers who challenge the promise of better health that the government had bestowed on their daughters.

Past, present, and future saturate this book, one of cultural and social transformation. The vignette of the mobile clinic, journeying from Bucharest to Roșiorii de Vede, includes several exoticizing stereotypes of Romania and eastern Europe: unlikely amalgams of rural traditionalism and futuristic postmodernity, poverty and conspicuous consumption, megalomaniacal architecture, subsistence agriculture, bankrupt postcommunist industries, Eastern Orthodox spirituality, idyllic landscapes, patriarchal divisions of labor and leisure time, nomadic Roma, stray dogs, broken roads, dust and dirt. When instrumentalized as part of a politics of representing otherness, these clichés irritate many Romanians, including me. However, in this book, I am not concerned with the ideological value of such representations. I am rather interested in their value as "*symptoms*, direct or mystified, of the true force of things" (Sahlins 1981,7). Like many other citizens witnessing the dismantling of the worlds in which they grew up, I attend to "the myriad sundry details of a vanished way of life" as "the only way to chase the catastrophe into the contours of the ordinary and try to tell a story" (Alexievich 2016, 7). I look through the lens of cultural and social transformation to describe "a world of vulnerability and unreasonable relationships" (White 2000, 5) in which most ordinary people dream of "getting by" (Kideckel 2008).

The book is divided into two parts. In part I, "Women's, Men's, and God's Will," I focus on ordinary people as subjects targeted for sexual and reproductive preventive care—Romanian women and men—and on the moralities that govern their sexual and reproductive lives. In part II, "Medicine and Its Moralities," I examine the structural forces that shape the provision of sexual and reproductive care in the context of postcommunist restructuring of state medicine, privatization of medical care, and the (re)emergence of inequitable forms of care. Each of the two parts of the book features a brief interlude summarizing government-led and, respectively, NGO-driven institutional developments regarding cervical cancer prevention in Romania.

The first two chapters provide the context to Romania's cervical cancer burden. I consider the historical trauma produced by brutally enforced reproductive policies and the alienation created by patriarchal relationships. Chapter 1, "We All Descend from Communism," is a tribute to history. I examine the political and cultural forces that have shaped Romanian women's reproductive health in the last seven decades, with a focus on the repressive communist pronatalist policies implemented between 1967 and 1989. To gauge the potential long-term side effects of past reproductive policies on women's health and well-being, I draw on the reproductive life history of Oana, one of my key research participants and a cervical cancer survivor. I show that the reproductive decisions that Oana and her peers faced as a result of being subjected to traumatic demographic and family policies in the past have left enduring legacies inscribed both symbolically and literally on present and future individual bodies.

Women are not the only ones impacted by reproductive policies. Using a mix of documentary and ethnographic sources, in chapter 2, "Reproductive Invisibility," I locate men within the historical, political, and cultural contexts of reproduction in communist and postcommunist Romania. I demonstrate how, by generating invisible men in the realm of reproduction, the communist- and postcommunist-enabled patriarchy has produced ripple effects on women's sexual and reproductive well-being. I also highlight the extent to which many women's lives are still shaped by patriarchal ideology and practice. That men are not held accountable for the reproductive consequences of their sexuality has important consequences regarding sexual and reproductive health promotion.

In chapter 3, "Beyond Rationalities," I take up suggestions from "nonsecular medical anthropology" (Whitmarsh and Roberts 2016) and examine the local moralities that shape the sexual and reproductive lives of women from Delcel. I look at how women mobilize lived religion as a decision-making resource in contexts of perceived reproductive vulnerability, when they lack support from both the state and their male partners. Entrusting health and especially prevention to

"God's will" provides a nonsecular rationale to their refusal of cervical screening and HPV vaccination.

In chapters 4, 5, and 6, I consider cervical cancer incidence and mortality in relation to the political economy of health care delivery, structural violence, and local forms of stratified reproduction. I highlight the ways in which emergent transformations in the provision of health care have shaped people's responses to state and private medicine, including their reactions to cervical cancer prevention programs. In chapter 4, "Dismantling Medicine," I use the theoretical distinction between "strategy" and "tactic" (De Certeau [1984] 2011) to scrutinize the impact of the recent strategic reforming of state medicine on Romanian women's tactics of accessing sexual and reproductive care. I investigate the ways citizens experience and conceptualize the emergent mutations in state-subsidized medicine with the idea that understanding people's reactions to these new regimes of public care provides us with yet another lens to understand the failure of state-driven cervical cancer prevention. I also explore some of the intergenerational differences and continuities in women's behaviors in seeking reproductive health and ponder their significance in changing understandings of state medicine.

In addition to postcommunist transformations of state medicine, the privatization of some sectors of health care brought about a multiplication of medical care delivery channels. In chapter 5, "The Other Hospital," I consider some of the ways in which changing ideas about sexual and reproductive care, including cervical cancer prevention, have been impacted by the possibility of accessing forms of care beyond state medicine. Exposed to the unprecedented choice between public and private reproductive medicine, some women struggle to produce new definitions of what counts as adequate care and to locate that care in specific institutions.

If chapter 3 is about the local moralities of sexuality and reproduction, chapter 6 mirrors those ideas by engaging with women's concerns with the moralities of sexual and reproductive health care. In chapter 6, "Locating Corruption," I show how cervical cancer prevention programs provided Romanians with the opportunity to use the idiom of corruption to locate ubiquitous yet volatile ideas about reproduction and to simultaneously express their conflicting perspectives on postcommunist medicine. The pervasive preoccupation with the moralities of reproductive care are responses to the uncertainties produced by both the dismantling of state medicine and the emergence of private medicine explored in the previous two chapters.

While I am concerned with cervical cancer prevention in particular historical and cultural circumstances, I conclude the book by pondering the relevance of small-scale results at transnational and global levels in a brief chapter titled "The Space between Informed and Non-Informed Refusal." My findings are relevant outside the Romanian context, as I highlight the factors that contribute to what experts dismiss as the "non-informed refusal" of medical intervention. Especially in the light of anti-vaccination controversies in the United States and beyond, I demonstrate the role that anthropology can play in tackling contemporary human challenges.

At the same time that the Renaşterea white and pink mobile clinic was traveling toward its destination to deliver preventive health services, some of its potential recipients from Roşiorii de Vede were driving in the reverse direction to Bucharest's public hospitals and private clinics in search of their own version of desired medical care.

The Cancer Within tells the story of this missed encounter between the providers of reproductive care and Romanian women.

PART 1 WOMEN'S, MEN'S, AND GOD'S WILL

1 • "WE ALL DESCEND FROM COMMUNISM"

My friend and I were only twenty-four, but both of us wished we were older, much older, so that we would not bear children anymore.

Oana, the woman who confesses to having once had such an unusual wish, stares at me intently. A peaceful early May dusk is falling as we chat in the backyard of her Roșiorii house, seated under sweet-scented lilac bushes. I look at Oana's face and notice that her lipstick—a rather garish shade of mauve—has bled into the fine lines surrounding her mouth. The intense color of her lips accentuates her crooked teeth. The look is not flattering. Oana recounts her life using animated words and penetrating images, and I cannot help looking at her with a mix of fascination and slight distaste. This embarrasses me: I am failing my goal to be an unbiased anthropologist.

More than forty years have passed since the times Oana invokes. Now in her late sixties, Oana, like many other Romanian women of her generation, has been participant and witness to seven decades of post–World War II history. Often interrupted by radical changes, her life has also been shaped by remarkable continuities. Born after the war, in a Romania that was forcibly abandoning a constitutional monarchy to become a Soviet political satellite, Oana grew up during the Stalinist purges of the 1950s. She briefly blossomed as a teenager during the 1960s political and cultural thaw, only to start her family shortly after the dictator Nicolae Ceaușescu promulgated strictly enforced pronatalist policies. Throughout the 1970s and 1980s, like most women of her generation, she struggled with the triple burden of motherhood, housekeeping, and a full-time career, in an era of reproductive rights restrictions and economic shortages. By the time Ceaușescu was ousted from power during the 1989 anti-communist bloodshed, Oana was premenopausal with grown-up children. Like many other Romanians, she spent the next two decades increasingly disenfranchised and disillusioned by the country's difficult transition to democracy and market economy.

When Romania joined the European Union (EU) in 2007, recently widowed and retired, Oana left the country for Italy. She worked in unskilled jobs for a few years, saving money. Back in Roșiorii, she renovated the house that she had inherited from her late husband's parents. Breaking with the local subsistence agriculture tradition of vegetable and potato gardens, Oana planted every strip of land surrounding her house with hundreds of tulips, lilies, begonias, and chrysanthemums. She wanted to have flowers blossom from early spring through late autumn. She covered the muddy alley between the street and the house entrance with an intricate design of gray paving and white mosaic, featuring a rather artless "2011"—the year the house renovation began. She converted an old pantry into a modern bathroom and had a water pressure system installed to pump water from a well into the kitchen and bathroom sewer. In her backyard, Oana planted a few white and purple lilac cuttings that she had received from a neighbor and set up a plastic table and chairs. A cozy, pleasant corner for herself. This is where she enjoyed her morning coffee and afternoon snacks, chatted with friends and neighbors, and occasionally had late summer dinners with visiting family members. This is where we chatted and gossiped and where I conducted my interviews with her. This is where, in a quiet evening of 2013, Oana sat in disbelief after learning that she had been diagnosed with cervical cancer.

If most of the other women with whom I talked were reserved during our early conversations, Oana was always eager to discuss sexuality, reproduction, and reproductive health issues. Looking at her life experiences through the lens of reproduction, it becomes apparent that—albeit historical circumstances kept changing—the underlying story of each decade of her life was essentially the same. Throughout Oana's life, Romanian women's reproductive rights were continuously set up against patriarchal-inspired informal and official agendas that repressed female sexuality while celebrating motherhood. The continuities in ordinary women's responses to these "many faces of patriarchy" (Miroiu 2002) are remarkable. Regardless of the changing political regimes of the last seven decades, Romanian women have resorted to recurring tactics to manage their reproduction.

This chapter is a tribute to history. I examine the political and cultural forces that have shaped women's reproductive rights and reproductive health under various regimes of patriarchy, from the traditional peasant family through the communist state paternalism to the contemporary redefining of gender roles. I employ Oana's "reproductive life history" (Inhorn 2012, 100) to convey the tangible ways in which reproductive policies become sites of cultural contestation for ordinary citizens. Attesting to the fact that, in contemporary Romania, "we all descend from communism" (Boia 2016, 201), the reproductive decisions that Oana and her peers faced when subjected to traumatic demographic and family policies in the past have not remained "in the past" (see also Anton 2009, 2014). The legacies of women's reproductive experiences are inscribed in the present and the future of individual bodies. As I highlight the systemic contingencies that have contributed to Romania's current cervical cancer crisis, I follow and untangle the complicated historical threads of family and reproductive policies.

Before further delving into Romania's recent history as witnessed and lived by Oana and her peers, I should note that, like other anthropologists, I am concerned with the moral and intellectual dilemmas that fieldwork generates. Weaving Oana's narrative into a broader chronicle of the historical traumas that I recount in this chapter is not without problems. How representative is Oana's life for an entire generation of Romanian women? To what extent do her particular reproductive experiences capture the lived realities of what reproduction might have entailed for millions of other women? Am I inadvertently reordering *post-festum* the timeline of Oana's life? Should we be concerned with the factual inaccuracies of some of her recollections? Like other anthropologists, I do not have an unequivocal answer to these questions. As one of my key study participants, Oana is at the same time ordinary and unique. Her life and reproductive experiences, while similar in significant ways to those of many other women born immediately after WWII, have often a particular poignancy because of her exceptional storytelling abilities. Also, Oana is one of the only five college-educated women among the forty-three who shared their stories with me. Her higher level of education sets her apart from most other women of Delcel but does not make her atypical. Oana's experiences, aspirations, and concerns overlap with those of the other Romanian women (Kligman 1998; Gal and Kligman 2000; Iepan 2005; Anton 2009, 2014; Miroiu and Dragomir 2010). Many of these women belong to a somewhat tragic generation: born too late to get a taste of the times that preceded the communist rule, yet too early to make it unscathed through the postcommunist transition. Their lives seem inescapably enclosed between the brackets of a never experienced *ex ante* and a perplexing *ex post*. Nevertheless, the lived realities of their existence under a repressive totalitarian regime transcend their time and speak about how "bodies remember" (Fassin 2007).

GROWING UP DURING THE OBSESSIVE DECADE

Oana recalls starting every day as a schoolchild singing in choir the Soviet anthem while looking at the photo-portrait of the Romanian Workers' Party secretary-general, which was hanging on the eastern wall of the classroom. That daily secular ritual was a reflection of postwar political and cultural transformations. The Romanian Communist Party (known as the Romanian Workers' Party between 1948 and 1965) was the sole leading political force of the country. Stalinism had been enforced as the state's official ideology. "The obsessive decade" (*obsedantul deceniu*)—as the 1948 to 1959 era was later known in Romanian historiography[1]—was a time of forcible political, social, and cultural change, marked by interdictions of civil rights, confiscation of private property, economic shortages, and political purges (Tismăneanu 2003; Boia 2016). Oana's own paternal grandfather had been arrested in the early 1950s, declared an "enemy of the nation," and sent to forced labor at the Danube-Black Sea Canal.

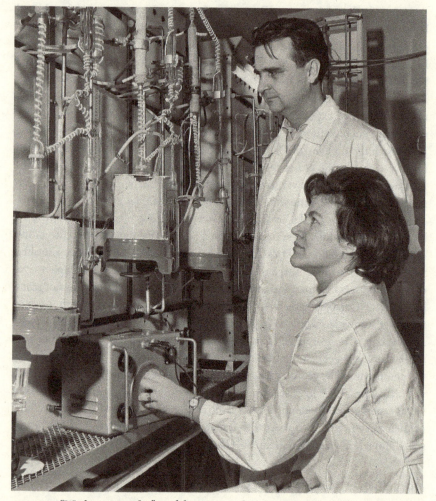

FIGURE 3. "Working comrades" in a laboratory, early 1960s. Reprinted with permission, courtesy of Minerva Photographic Archives of the Minerva Cultural Association, Cluj, Romania.

Following the Soviet Union's lead, the Romanian Communist Party undertook a vast modernization mission. A crucial part of this project was applying Lenin's vision about freeing women from "the pettiness of domestic life" by integrating them into the active workforce (Gal and Kligman 2000; Du Plessix Gray 1989). In 1946 Romanian women were granted suffrage and were recognized as "full, capable citizens" (Roman 2001, 53), and from 1948, the party further promoted the emancipation of women. For the first time in Romania's history, women joined men in the labor force as "working comrades" (figure 3), in the education system as "school comrades," and in family as "life comrades" (Miroiu 2010). This politics of affirmative action brought about the de-feminization of women. The iconography of realist socialism abounds in representations of androgynous-looking working women devoutly operating hard industry machines, shoulder to shoulder with their male "working comrades" (Buchel and Carmine 2008).

The new regime claimed that it had discontinued traditional gender roles. However, it did perpetuate patriarchy by silencing women's sexuality and promoting "an egalitarianism flavored with state patriarchy" (Miroiu 2010, 582; David and Băban 1996; Anton 2009). While state paternalism affected both men and women, we can grasp the full extent to which the state was interfering with the lives of its citizens when we examine reproductive policies. In response to demographic concerns over the future of the workforce, in 1948, following Soviet directives, the Romanian communist government outlawed abortion (which had been partly liberalized since 1937). Under declining economic conditions, with postwar food shortages amplified by the most severe drought of the twentieth century, women had increasingly used abortion to control their fertility. However, abortion as a method of birth control was not new. In a preeminently rural patriarchal society that valued high fertility and did not endorse contraception, women had been using abortion as birth control for generations. Following the 1948 criminalization of abortion, Romanian women continued to clandestinely terminate unwanted pregnancies.

The obsessive decade was eventful. Following Stalin's death in 1953, political purges gradually waned in the Soviet Union and its political satellites, including Romania. In 1956, the new Soviet leader, Nikita Khrushchev, delivered "the secret speech," which marked the beginning of "the Thaw"—an era of amends to previous repression. For Romanian women, one consequence of the new political climate was the 1957 legalization of abortion. Following again the Soviet lead, other eastern European countries from the communist bloc (such as Bulgaria, Hungary, Poland, and Czechoslovakia) also decriminalized abortion in 1957. Several ideological and practical factors contributed to this. First, since the local production of contraceptives was almost nonexistent in communist countries, modern contraception was imported from "the West." Making abortion legal and affordable aimed at curbing women's reliance on capitalist-produced contraception (Vassilev 1999). Second, legal abortion was an instrument of biopolitics and state reproductive surveillance, as it reduced the number of unrecorded back-alley abortions. Finally, in an officially atheistic society, abortion became less morally stigmatized (David 1999).

Then, Oana was too young to be concerned with reproductive policies. Her most poignant childhood memory is nevertheless significant of the world of alienating repression in which she grew up. This is how she remembers a midsummer night in 1955:

One evening, my father took me to the railway station. Grandpa [had been released from forced labor and] was returning home. We waited for the train on the dimly lit platform. Finally, the train entered the station with a long whistling. People started to get out from the train and leave the station until the platform got empty. No sight of Grandpa.

Turning her head to one side and then to another, Oana continues:

My father and I looked around, to the left, to the right ... nothing. Suddenly, a frail shadow emerged from the dark and an old [bătrân] and emaciated [slab] man stopped in front of us.

Oana lengthens the vowels in bătrân and slab in a wailing sounding sentence.

My father and I both stared at the strange apparition just to realize, on a second glance, that it was Grandpa, unrecognizably worn out.

TEENAGER IN THE TIME OF THE THAW

From the 1960s, Oana recalls the miraculous sensation she experienced when she wore, for the first time, nylon pantyhose, and the Beatles versus Rolling Stones wars that divided her high school classmates. Long forgotten was the Soviet anthem! In the aftermath of the post-Stalinist thaw, economic conditions improved and the cultural climate changed. With "a surrogacy of prosperity ... and a simulacrum of freedom" (Boia 2016, 101), Romania became one of the most liberal countries from the eastern communist bloc (figure 4). Women continued to have legal access to cheap and safe abortions. In the early 1960s, it was not uncommon to see in Bucharest women waiting in long lines in front of state-owned abortion clinics for the procedure that cost the equivalent of less than $2 (Kligman 1998, 47). Yet, state control over reproduction was soon about to take a turn for the worse.

STARTING A FAMILY UNDER PRONATALISM

During the first two decades of communist rule, motherhood was not part of the official vision for women as loyal citizens. Yet, in 1966, reproduction emerged as a site of extreme state control when the adoption of Decree 770 restrained women's rights to interrupt the course of a pregnancy (David and Băban 1996; Kligman 1998; Băban 1999; Miroiu 2010; Jinga 2015).[2] The rise to power of Nicolae Ceaușescu—who became the Romanian Communist Party's leader in 1965, and one of the most authoritarian dictators of modern times—marked the separation of Romanian communism from its Soviet source. Ceaușescu's ambition was to create an original, ethnic-based version of socialism, later labeled "national-communism" (Tismăneanu 2003). He was preoccupied with population growth because his megalomaniacal projects needed a large workforce.

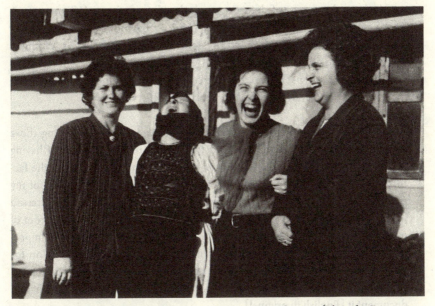

FIGURE 4. Enjoying the Thaw. Romanian women in the mid-1960s. (Photo by Răzvan Givulescu, reprinted with permission.)

Under Ceaușescu's leadership, the regime acted both supportively and coercively to produce an increase in birth rates. On the one hand, the state offered social incentives to high natality, such as state-financed daycare and preschools, shorter work schedules for breastfeeding mothers, paid benefits for new mothers, and allocations for children (Băban 1999; Keil and Andreescu 1999). While communist propaganda broadcast social programs as evidence of a caring welfare state, the reality was that the paternalist state promoted family policies aimed at appropriating children—"the future of the country"—through early institutionalization. On the other hand, state authorities resorted to interdictions and constraints to stimulate natality. Under Ceaușescu's dictatorship, Romania had one of the strictest pronatalist policies in the world (David and Băban 1996; Kligman 1998; Keil and Andreescu 1999; Doboș, Jinga, and Soare 2010; Jinga et al. 2011). The Soviet Union and other eastern European communist countries had also implemented pronatalist policies in the late 1960s, but these pronatalist regimes were gradually relaxed and women were granted access to contraception during the 1970s and 1980s. Unlike its communist neighbors, Romania continued to pursue "a rigidly enforced pronatalist policy, banning the importation of contraceptives, strictly prohibiting most abortions, and imposing a tax on childless couples" (Băban 1999, 191). Furthermore, most women were subjected to periodical mandatory gynecological exams in the workplace, where they could be more easily surveyed. Sometimes, these exams included Pap tests, used as a cover for the real purpose of detecting undeclared pregnancies (Kligman 1998, 154). When a woman was suspected of seeking or having sought a back-alley abortion, a prosecutor was appointed to attend her medical checkups. Women's wombs had become state property.

One male gynecologist featured in a documentary by filmmaker Florin Iepan (2005) recalled performing medical controls in a factory:

> In the factory the women were caught, they had no escape.... During those times, they didn't like to go to the doctor for that reason [the risk of having an unwanted pregnancy exposed before trying to terminate it], but in the factory they could be forced to do it. In two hours—and I am not proud of my performance—I had seen between forty and sixty women.... They got undressed in the back. They were given no gowns, they came completely naked in front of me, going in, on two tables. [It] was like a grotesque ballet. And what was important for the authorities [was] their last menstruation. It was an obsession for them, for the Communist Party, the last period of the women. And if I founded [sic] that one of them was pregnant, [that she] had the uterus enlarged I had to document it [English in original].

A former worker in a textile factory remembered the way she and her workmates were summoned to mandatory controls:

> The foreman would come next to the weaving looms and say: *You have to go to the consultation room.* Then he would turn to the girl next to me or the one in front of me, because there were several girls that had to be checked. Maybe ten, or twenty, or thirty girls. If we hadn't gone, they would have had us face the Communist Party and I don't know what would have happened to us there. We were so afraid of the Party.... (Iepan 2005; see also Gal and Kligman 2000, 232)

In 1978, midwifery was discontinued as a medical profession. Midwifery training was assimilated with nursing, and former midwives were placed under the direct supervision of OB-GYNs. As nurses, the new midwives did not receive specialized obstetrical training anymore (Vlădescu 2009). As paradoxical as it may seem, given the strong pronatalist orientation of the government, the termination of midwifery was an attempt to tighten state control over reproduction by limiting the professional autonomy of medical workers who were seen to be the closest to pregnant women. Traditionally, rural midwives (sage women without formal medical training) were known for both facilitating births and providing abortions. Starting from the 1950s, midwives who received formal medical education became licensed health care professionals. To earn an income on the market of clandestine abortions, under pronatalism midwives capitalized on their reputation as birth preventers rather than birth facilitators. By eliminating midwives, the communist state attempted to delegitimize their role in performing back-alley abortions. The lack of midwives amplified the "technocratic" birthing experience (exclusively hospital based, with only lithotomy position) for women, especially since most OB-GYNs were men (Miroiu and Dragomir 2010). The cessation of midwifery provides an example of the contradictions that defined the totalitarian state. By limiting the number of medical workers specifically trained to assist births, the state undermined its own long-term interests of increasing natality while also compromising its ideological claims about safe reproduction.

It was under these circumstances that Oana started a family in the early 1970s. She married her college sweetheart, a construction engineer she had met while studying at the Polytechnic University in Bucharest. First, they rented a studio apartment in Roșiorii de Vede. Once their first child was born, they moved into a two-bedroom apartment that they secured through the welfare program for the employees of the factory where they both worked. Young Oana's wish to be past her prime—as I quoted in the opening of the chapter—was part of her recalling the hardships of sexual life in Ceaușescu's Romania. As a young wife, she had almost no access to modern contraception, which was accessible only through informal connections on the black market. Oral contraceptives, brought into the country from Hungary and Yugoslavia, were surreptitiously advertised by word-of-mouth as *antibebi* (from the English "anti-baby"). Low-quality condoms imported from China could sporadically be found in some pharmacies, but they were usually available under-the-table, with women learning of them through personal connections. Oana and other women used natural contraception, such as the calendar, withdrawal, or douching. The scarcity of contraceptive resources did not deter women from engaging in sexual relations. Oana and some of her peers who shared their reproductive life histories with me invoked the loneliness of being a young wife in a country whose strong roots in rural patriarchy deemed sexuality in general—and female sexuality in particular—as inappropriate topics for conversations. Neither their husbands nor their mothers-in-law, and often not even their own mothers, would consider contraception a topic for open discussion. Hence, young Oana and others looked forward to menopause (see also David and Băban 1996, 242; Gal and Kligman 2000, 232; Miroiu and Dragomir 2010).

Following the adoption of Decree 770, birth rates and total fertility rates doubled from 1966 to 1968.[3] The children born in 1967 and the subsequent three years are sarcastically known in Romania as "the children of the decree" (*decrețeii*) or "Ceaușescu's kids" (*ceaușeii*). Starting with 1973, birth rates slowly but steadily decreased again, reaching the pre-1966 levels by the end of the 1980s (Kligman 1998; Keil and Andreescu 1999; Iepan 2005). In response to the state's brutal intrusion into their reproductive lives, women used birth control ranging from sexual abstinence and natural contraception to under-the-table modern contraception and back-alley abortions. In retrospect, many women who lived their reproductive years during Ceaușescu regime identified sexuality and its risks as the main cause for personal stress. They remembered feeling disempowered and humiliated because they lacked control over their sexuality, their bodies, and their own—sometimes unwanted—children's existence (Kligman 1995, 1998; Miroiu 2010). Some recalled how "a couple's life was terrorized by this detail: twelve times a year you might have a baby," and how, fearing conception, "[sexual intercourse] was an event that happened rarely, only programmed" (Iepan 2005).

One of Oana's neighbors from Delcel, retired factory inspector Veturia, eighty-seven years old, hinted at having had a double-digit number of abortions (that conversation is recalled in chapter 3). She summarized her perceived lack of reproductive alternatives: "We were supposed to just welcome them [the children] all." As for Oana, she colorfully captures the dehumanizing experience of forced reproduction: "I was feeling like a breeding cow."

THE ABORTION DIARIES

One of the main unintended consequences of Decree 770 was the increase in back-alley abortions. Between 1966 and 1989, the number of clandestine abortions skyrocketed, reaching the proportions of a lucrative industry led by backdoor abortion providers (Kligman 1998; Stan and Turcescu 2007; Miroiu 2010).[4] Abortions were often performed in apartments, kitchens, bathrooms, or pantries, under nonsterile conditions.[5] Abortion providers and pregnant women exchanged minimal mutual information to prevent identification if caught by the authorities. Abortion seekers often used passwords to enter abortion sites. Many of the providers had no formal medical training and used either improvised devices or folk medicine remedies believed to have abortifacient effects. Others relied on basic allopathic medicine knowledge and inserted a catheter into the uterus. The demand for clandestine abortions was high, and the legal consequences of being caught while having or performing an abortion were very serious, with imprisonment for both provider and client. This is why most abortion providers set high prices for the procedure.[6] However, some of them practiced differential tariffs, based on a pregnant woman's income (Iepan 2005). Despite legal and medical risks and high costs, many women resorted to abortions, especially during the severe economic shortages of the 1980s.[7] Oana already had two children when she found herself pregnant again. This is how she recalls her attempt to terminate the pregnancy:

It happened some time in '75 or '76. My mom had this acquaintance—a pharmacist—and she provided me with a full battery of injections . . . to break up the embryo into pieces. And I took [the injections] and then I waited and waited, and eventually I started to bleed, and I had a huge hemorrhage. I called the ambulance. They came with an old, broken car, completely empty.

We should not let Oana's matter-of-fact tone obfuscate the grim reality of the scene she describes: A heavily bleeding woman is given an emergency ride to the hospital in a "completely empty" ambulance. It is significant that, decades later, she still finds a way to weave this detail into her story. Oana's first clandestine abortion reveals the contrast between the resourcefulness activated through her network of informal connections and the shortages of official state medicine. Once at the hospital, Oana tried to frame the abortion as a miscarriage:

The doctor asked me what had happened. I lied that we had moved, and I had carried heavy furniture. And I also lied about the date of the last menstruation. I declared it much later, so I could claim that I was ignorant of my condition. I was keeping a real and a make-believe evidence of my menstruations in two small notebooks. That proved helpful for the couple of times when I had to tamper [with that record] and make up different [last menstruation] dates. At the hospital they gave me a vacuum aspiration and let me go without further questioning.

In her interactions with the medical staff at the hospital, Oana was deliberately duplicitous. She answered deceitfully to the doctor's interrogation. By doing so, she violated medicine's normative expectations that bound the patient to truthful cooperation with the medical provider during anamnesis and clinical examination. Oana's deception could have potentially exposed her to further risks. Yet Oana had no choice but to hide the truth, knowing that the confidentiality of the clinical exam was not granted. Medical workers, especially OB-GYNs, were subjected to political surveillance. The whole medical encounter became a masquerade marred by mistrust.

But what was the purpose of the perplexing practice of keeping two distinct records of the last menstruation? As revealed in many accounts about the pronatalist regime, recording the date of a woman's last menstruation was of paramount concern to the state authorities. The date was used as a biopolitical instrument of surveillance to detect and record undeclared pregnancies (Kligman 1998; Iepan 2005). By keeping both real and fake evidence of her last menstruation, Oana demonstrated that she was aware of the political importance of recording practices, which she managed to outpower through fake reporting. The fabricated last menstruation date was part of Oana's arsenal of "the weapons of the weak" (Scott 1985). The two divergent records that she kept embody the contrast between the intimate, resourceful, and authentic private existence of ordinary women and their vulnerable, fraught, and deceptive public performance. Oana's and other women's recollections of their reproductive experiences during pronatalism demonstrate that the medical examination became not only a locus of power struggle but also a site for embracing or resisting state policies. Some medical providers would internalize state paternalism and would subject their patients to patriarchal forms of violence—such as blaming women for the alleged pleasures of having sex or submitting them to humiliating bodily postures during the medical checkup (Kligman 1998; Pârvulescu 2015). There are, however, countless stories about doctors' solidarity with women seeking illegal abortions. Oana's account of her second underground abortion reveals precisely the shifting nature of the power relations between doctors and women.

Toward the end of 1970s, Oana attempted to get another clandestine abortion. She remembers:

> The second time was worse. There were more restrictions. Many obstetricians and women had been jailed for illegal abortions. So, out of the blue, I craved meatballs. I started to worry . . . and of course I was [pregnant] again.
>
> I took those injections again, but nothing happened, time passed, nothing [happened]. Then, a friend of my sister-in-law referred me to a doctor who was just part-time affiliated with the maternity hospital. I went to the ambulatory room of the hospital. The doctor tried something, but with no result. A few days later, a relative of my sister-in-law's friend arranged things with a medical nurse. That nurse and I, we still see each other on the street from time to time, but we both pretend that we don't know each other anymore. So I went to my sister-in-law's relative's place, at her home, and there the nurse inserted a catheter. And— miracle!—I started to bleed heavily, with clots.

Oana was able to mobilize even more private resources than for her first back-alley abortion. A whole "whisper network" of family members, friends, acquaintances, and strangers were involved in these clandestine practices, including the part-time affiliated doctor who tried to perform an illegal abortion inside the state hospital. I will briefly return to this episode in chapter 2, where I analyze the roles from a gendered perspective. For now, I focus on this doctor's ability to bridge the hidden and the visible realms of medicine. Oana's story shows that co-participating in illegal reproductive practices entails human solidarity but also long-term estrangement within these informal networks. Oana continued her story on a disconcerting tragicomic note, with her duplicitous attempt to frame again the abortion as a miscarriage:

> I ran to the hospital, and they put me in the same room with other heavily bleeding women—they were all suspected of having tried to terminate their pregnancies. Later on, they brought in another one, a young one, [she was] a history teacher, she was half dead from bleeding, poor thing, but they managed to save her.

And then the frog episode followed. They used our urine on frogs in the lab [to detect pregnancy]. And here comes one nurse—an ugly, unlikable face—and she comes from the lab into our room: *Who is Oana M.?* I stand up and she goes: *Your frog died!*

Oana throws her head back, laughing hard, before resuming:

Of course, the frog died, I thought, after all the poison cocktail I injected into myself. . . . And then the doctor came in and I showed him the bleeding. Of course, again: *What did you do? When was the last menstruation?* He saw the blood clots and scheduled me for a vacuum aspiration.

"The frog episode" unveils self-irony in Oana's strategy to cope with the repressive character of clinical examinations and care, but it also gives us another glimpse into the extent to which Romanian hospitals lacked modern medical resources during communism. Known also as the frog test, the Galli-Mainini test consist of "injecting a small amount of urine from a woman who suspects she is pregnant into the dorsal lymph sack of a male frog. If the woman is pregnant, the pregnancy hormone present in her urine will cause the frog to produce sperm, easily seen under a microscope, within three hours."[8] The test, once widely used worldwide from the 1940s, was abandoned in most countries by the 1960s when immunological tests became available. However, through to the late 1970s and early 1980s, it was still used in underresourced Romanian hospitals.

Oana's account reveals biopolitics in action. All women who come to the clinic with severe vaginal hemorrhage are placed in the same room. Extending political surveillance procedures, the hospital's screening practices create new categories of patients. Women's symptomatology makes them potential criminals. The waiting room becomes a sort of agonizing purgatory for these women, as their future—freedom or jail time, life or death—is decided through political action rather than medical expertise, as shown in the last episode of Oana's abortion story:

Finally, I was brought into the surgery room, I [was] laid on the table and there was a man right there, not a doctor, a civilian. He called *secu* [Securitate, the secret police] on the phone. *We have here a patient, heavily bleeding, with clots, we believe that the embryo is compromised. We cannot keep her pregnancy, so we ask permission to give her a vacuum aspiration.* Only after *secu* agreed, they proceeded with the aspiration.

The application rules of Decree 770, issued in January 1974, stipulated that for each woman diagnosed with incomplete abortion, prior to proceeding to the vacuum aspiration of the uterus, the OB-GYN had the obligation to call either the local prosecutor's office during regular hours or the local police department for after-hours interventions (Doboş, Jinga, and Soare 2010, 342). Given these regulations, Oana's account is inaccurate. Most likely, a phone call was made from the surgery room, but, according to official procedures, the doctor—and not someone else—would have called the regular police, not the secret police. These inexactitudes may be due either to the clinic's bending of the rules or to Oana's misunderstanding of the communication procedures during a stressful moment of her life, or simply to her memory failing to recover all the details four decades after the events she narrated. Prosecutors would often come to maternity hospitals to document cases of illegal abortions (Kligman 1998; David and Băban 1996). Also, in Ceauşescu's Romania, all institutions had an affiliated representative from *Securitate*. To ordinary citizens, the regular police (known as *miliţie*) and the political police represented similar faces of repression. Oana's claim that "a civilian" (maybe a prosecutor? maybe the *Securitate* affiliate of the hospital?) called the political police to inform them about the imminent vacuum aspiration is plausible. But it is not important to establish the absolute truth of this story. What makes Oana's account significant are precisely its inaccuracies (see also White 2000). In her telling of this abortion, the enigmatic figure of the "civilian" represents state authority, while the secret police assumes the decision-making role. Her recollection illustrates the relational—rather than the factual—character of post-communist remembrance (Anton 2009, 2014). Oana's story features the quintessential mechanisms of power and control under dictatorship. Reproductive care takes place at the intersection between state surveillance—literally embodied in the persona of "the civilian"—and political repression in the form of the discretionary voice at the other end of the line. Medical expertise is relegated to a marginal means to achieve political ends. Oana's story illustrates her understanding of reproductive care as politically managed and of state medicine as irrelevant.

There is, nevertheless, a last twist to this chilling narrative. According to Oana, it turns out that some of the women with whom she shared the waiting room—all of them suspected of having tried to have a clandestine abortion—were in fact *secu* officers' wives. The pronatalist regime did not spare anyone.

DARK AND DIM STORIES FROM THE GOLDEN AGE

The contrast between the grim realities of everyday life and the regime's claims of magnificence reached an ironic culmination in the mid-1980s, when Ceauşescu era was officially rebranded as "the Golden Age" (*epoca de aur*). Described by the communist propaganda as a glorious time in Romania's history, the 1980s were in reality better known for the extravagant cult of personality of Ceauşescu and his wife, restrictions of civil liberties, daily power outages, extreme shortages of most consumption goods, and the rationing of staple foods. Informal economy exchanges became crucial to the very survival of ordinary citizens. Women seemed to be particularly affected by the harsh life conditions of the Golden Age. In addition to having their reproductive rights restricted, they faced the much discussed "triple burden" of being full-time workers, mothers, and wives (Kligman 1998; Jinga 2015). Oana remembers the following episode from the 1980s:

> One winter evening, I was returning home from work. I had picked up my daughter from her math tutor and we had queued together in a long line to get oranges. It was late when we walked to our neighborhood. Pitch dark on the streets. Pitch dark inside apartment buildings. As we came close to home, a drunkard started making after us. He was hissing and grunting behind us on the sidewalk. I grabbed my daughter's hand and we both started to run, the bag of oranges in my other hand and my shoulder bag clumsy sitting across my coat. We were running together in that pitch black. . . .

The image of the mother and her daughter running together in the darkness could be an allegory of the condition of Romanian women in the 1980s: living in fear, uncertainty, and isolation, in cold and darkness, with no escape in sight. The statement that I heard time and again from the women of Roșiorii in reference to the Golden Age captured precisely this traumatic foreshortening of the future: "Those were not good times to have more children" (see also David and Băban 1996, 242).

Unsurprisingly, there are no ethnographic accounts from the late communist era featuring positive memories of women's reproductive experiences. Yet, among the women from Delcel, a handful seemed to have favorable recollections of their pregnancies, childbirth, and maternity years during pronatalism. Among them were Tereza, Ramona, and Sorana, all of whom struggled with infertility for years before conceiving their babies. Pressured to report high birth rates, OB-GYNs kept women who had fertility issues under strict clinical observation during pregnancies to ensure live births. While these women acknowledged the unreasonable power relations that bound doctors and patients to forms of biopolitical repression, they were nevertheless grateful that the workings of an authoritarian regime granted them successful pregnancy outcomes.

One of Oana's neighbors, Tereza, is fifty-seven years old and the proud mother of a twenty-six-year-old daughter who lives in Bucharest with her husband. As a young wife, Tereza struggled with fertility problems for years. In her twenties, she suffered two second trimester miscarriages (at four and a half and six months, respectively) and was diagnosed with uterine fibromatosis. She underwent several series of hormonal treatments. Unlike most women who admitted having had occasionally employed folk medicine remedies for reproductive ailments, Tereza is adamant in endorsing the benefits of biomedical treatment, and she dismisses "old women's remedies." In the mid-1980s, Tereza, then in her early thirties, found herself pregnant again. Her OB-GYN kept her under firm clinical observation for much of her pregnancy. She spent several weeks as a patient in the high-risk pregnancy quarter of the maternity hospital and was repeatedly subjected to various medical checkups, including pelvic exams and blood and urine analyses—all free of charge. Tereza was content with the overmedicalization of her condition because it appeased her fears of losing yet another baby. Between the fifth and the seventh month of her pregnancy, the fetus appeared to be stuck in a breech position. According to Tereza, this prompted her OB-GYN to decide on an early C-section delivery at around the twenty-eighth week of her pregnancy. Eventually, Tereza entered into labor just days before the scheduled C-section, and in a matter of a few hours, she gave birth without surgical intervention to a premature but healthy baby girl at 3.9 pounds and 15 inches.

Postpartum, Tereza and the baby remained hospitalized for four weeks; the baby was kept in an incubator in the neonatal intensive care unit (NICU) until she reached 5.5 pounds. An official birth certificate was issued ten days after the birth. As she was checking on her baby several times a day, Tereza started to compare her own newborn with another premature baby from the NICU who was born the same day and was placed in the next incubator. The other baby belonged to a mother who already had three children. The high birth rank of that newborn prompted Tereza to assume that the baby was in fact "a child of the decree"—a child born because the mother was unable to avoid the pregnancy or to secure a back-alley abortion once pregnant. Noticing that the other baby was gaining weight at a faster rate than her own, Tereza recalls standing next to the other baby's incubator and scolding her, half-jokingly: "What are you doing, baby? Why do you keep growing when your mother doesn't even want you? Why doesn't my baby girl, whom I wanted so much, grow as fast as you do?"

Like Tereza, Ramona, age 49, had to undertake fertility treatments to finally see her reproductive desires realized. An accountant holding a BA diploma, she married in the late 1970s with the intention of conceiving as soon as possible. Yet, three years into her marriage, Ramona had not succeeded in becoming pregnant. She was diagnosed with endometriosis and started fertility treatments. Three more years later, she found herself pregnant. She spent months in the hospital under medication. She gave birth to a premature baby girl weighing 4 pounds, who received an Apgar 7 because she was born with the umbilical cord around her neck and did not cry. The newborn was placed in the incubator in the NICU for about three weeks, but both mother and baby were released when the baby reached 5 pounds (instead of the standard of 5.5), with the provision that the neonatal doctor would come and visit them at home for the next couples of months. In Ramona's case, it took twenty-one days for the baby's official birth certificate to be issued. Worried about the fragility of her baby, Ramona made extensive use of informal contributions to the neonatal medical staff, with the understanding that this would secure better care for her baby. Because of the baby's prematurity, Ramona was granted privileged access to powdered milk, a rare commodity in the mid-1980s. Like Tereza, she recalls with appreciation the workings of the Ceaușescu era medical system. Even though she felt compelled to make informal contributions in exchange for privileged care for her baby, Ramona credits her reproductive success to the presumably increased standards of care for pregnant women and premature babies implemented by the pronatalist regime.

Sorana, an accountant with a high school diploma, was another woman from Roșiorii de Vede who shared with me her struggles to conceive during the 1980s, as a young wife in her early twenties. She claims having had a first trimester miscarriage, but she never went to the hospital or the dispensary, either to report the pregnancy or to diagnose the miscarriage. She became suspicious of her pregnant condition when she realized that the smell of homemade plum brandy, which she used to find pleasant, was suddenly making her nauseous. By the time her period was about three weeks late, she disclosed the news to her sister-in-law, who lived nearby. Days later, she had an abundant hemorrhage with blood clots, but, at her sister-in-law's advice, she did not take the day off from her workplace, dreading that her absence would arouse suspicions of an attempted clandestine abortion. The bleeding eventually stopped without further complications. Six months later, Sorana reported to the local dispensary with sharp abdominal pains. She was referred to an OB-GYN, diagnosed with ectopic pregnancy, and given emergency surgery in the local municipal hospital. Four years and numerous fertility treatments later, Sorana found herself pregnant again. Like Tereza and Ramona, she was closely monitored in both the local dispensary and the hospital to ensure a successful pregnancy. During a routine checkup at seven months, Sorana's cervix was found dilated. She was immediately hospitalized and bedbound and was administered medication aimed at preventing uterine contractions for the next few days. Nevertheless, Sorana started having labor pains. An emergency C-section was performed. Her baby girl was premature and weighed only 4 pounds; she was placed in an NICU incubator for a month. Mother and daughter were released from the hospital once the baby reached 5.5 pounds. Once again, the official birth certificate was issued with a ten-day postpartum delay. While Tereza and Sorana did not get pregnant again after giving birth to their unique offspring, Ramona had another pregnancy in 1989, but given the increased economic difficulties her family was facing, she sought a back-alley abortion.

It is hard to assess how typical these women's recollections are. They make up only 7 percent of the women who shared their reproductive life histories with me. However, these three cases were chosen "by virtue of their intrinsic interest"

(Elman, Gerring, and Mahoney 2016, 377) since Tereza, Ramona, and Sorana were the only ones who had personally fought infertility during a time when giving birth was also a matter of the most heightened political concern. Unlike all the other women from Delcel, all three have strikingly positive recollections of their experience of giving birth during the late communist years and saw themselves as privileged recipients of reproductive care under the pronatalist regime. They also tended to assume that their own reproductive aspirations converged with government politics of increasing birth rates, even though parental desires for actual babies were quite different from the regime's purely statistical demographic ambitions. While doctors were under pressure to report constant increases in the number of live births, there were in fact no normative forms of care specifically targeting women suffering from infertility. Even Ramona's truly privileged access to powdered milk was actually meant to enhance her postpartum productivity (by allowing her to resume work as soon as possible after birth) and had little to do with her premature baby and even less with her fertility struggles.

Notwithstanding their uncommon character, Tereza, Ramona, and Sorana all had reproductive life histories of fighting infertility during the pronatalist years, and their experiences can help us reach a more nuanced understanding of the politics of reproduction during the Golden Age in at least two distinct ways. These stories reveal the intricate ways in which different types of perceived reproductive vulnerability were linked to each other rather than experienced in an individual, atomistic way. Through an analysis of these cases, we can further explore reproductive vulnerability as an essentially intersubjective notion. Tereza's discursive performance of rhetorically and reproachfully addressing the other premature newborn in the NICU may seem strange. Yet this episode encapsulates the ways in which apparently opposite forms of reproductive vulnerability (respectively, infertility and unwanted fertility) were interconnected and mutually amplified during pronatalism. For the women struggling with infertility, the strenuous desire to reproduce was intensified by their awareness of their peers' struggles with unwelcome fertility produced by the restriction of reproductive rights. Recall Tereza's scolding of the presumably unwanted newborn. Similarly, Sorana's miscarriage episode shows that seemingly unrelated forms of reproductive vulnerability were "communicable" under a regime of bodily surveillance. Sorana did not allow herself to fully experience the grief, the discomfort, and the subsequent recovery time following her pregnancy loss, for fear of being misidentified as someone who had attempted a clandestine abortion.

These women's stories give us a particular glimpse into the inner workings of the pronatalist regime, especially its recording and reporting practices. Given their intensive socialization into the values and language of state medicine, all three women were preoccupied with normative newborn bodies and punctuated their recollections with numbers (length and weight of the baby, baby's weight gain, days spent in the NICU). However, as demonstrated in Ramona's case and her baby being released from the hospital before reaching 5.5 pounds, standards were not strictly enforced; rules could be bent, provided that medical surveillance was continued outside the hospital. Although the stories of Tereza, Ramona, and Sorana have happy endings, there is a dark underside to their memories that deepens our understanding of the actual reproductive experiences that the demographic ambitions of Ceauşescu regime would produce. Because their babies were premature, official birth certificates were issued with considerable delay, only after it became apparent that the babies would survive. During my time in Roşiorii de Vede, I also collected three more stories from mothers who, without fighting infertility, had given birth to premature babies shortly before 1989. They also had to wait between ten and twenty-one days for their baby's birth certificates to be issued (see also Băban 2000, 228). One gynecologist who practiced in the 1980s told me that some doctors reported the cases of premature infant death as stillbirths, in order to avoid the medical and legal investigations and sanctions that usually followed a newborn's death (personal communication, November 2009, with Dr. C. T.). Counting the death of an infant (premature or not) as a stillbirth lowered the official rates of infant mortality—a globally recognized indicator of public health effectiveness. By tacitly encouraging skewed reporting practices, the communist state propaganda promoted a prosperous image of the regime. It appears that, by 1988, the registration of live births was routinely delayed to adjust infant mortality rates. A physician explained to anthropologist Gail Kligman that "if you are not registered alive, then you are not registered dead either" (1998, 220). We can reasonably assume that some deceased newborns never existed officially because of such recording and reporting practices. None of the women from Delcel who shared their reproductive life histories with me confessed to having experienced neonatal death during the pronatalist years. Nevertheless, along with the accounts of women like Oana, who struggled with unwanted fertility, the stories of those who fought infertility complete the picture of the political mechanisms of reproduction surveillance. During the late communist era, false reporting plagued not only reproduction and medical care but virtually all venues of social, cultural, and economic life. To give just one example, the reported wheat harvests were so absurdly exaggerated that they would defy the physical laws of the maximal number of wheat ears that could grow on a given surface (Boia 2016, 143–144). By the end of the 1980s, Romania was gradually becoming an alienating propaganda bubble that was about to burst soon.

MENOPAUSE AND REVOLUTION

In December 1989, Ceauşescu's national communist regime was overthrown following a violent mass revolt. The dictator and his wife were executed after a summary lawsuit. Like many other Romanians, Oana talks about "the Revolution," evoking the awe, fear, and uncertainty of watching the bloodshed live on TV but also the excitement for a new future. As Romania became a democratic country literally overnight, political changes were abrupt and dramatic. The criminalization of abortion was repealed by a decree of the new political authority on December 26, one day after Ceaușescu's death. Unless a woman's life was endangered, abortion remained illegal only after fourteen gestational weeks (chapter IV, article 201, New Criminal Code 2016). Ironically, as one of the first laws to be adopted under a democratic regime, the legalization of abortion passed without any public debate. At that time, no one challenged the new law—not even the Romanian Orthodox Church—because for most Romanians, the pronatalist policy epitomized the oppressiveness of the communist state (Durandin and Petre 2010; Johnson, Horga, and Fajans 2004). As of 2021, there are no legal sanctions against women seeking clandestine abortions, but the 2016 Criminal Code stipulates punishments for abortion providers who have no medical training or perform abortions outside accredited medical institutions. For Oana personally, these changes came too late, as she was already perimenopausal in the early 1990s. For the following two decades, along with millions of Romanians, Oana got busy "getting by in postsocialist Romania" (Kideckel 2008).

The decriminalization of abortion was an important step toward freeing women from state control, even if it did not get rid entirely of patriarchy (Roman 2003; Miroiu 2002, 2010; Durandin and Petre 2010). However, women in need of safe abortions now face new structural barriers, such as financial costs, lack of transportation, and childcare. These are particularly true for women from remote or rural areas. In public hospitals, abortions are relatively inexpensive (the equivalent of $80 to $100 in 2021), but the quality of care is often very poor, with laxly enforced hygiene standards, worn-out infrastructure, and obsolete abortion procedures. Abortion in state hospitals are reportedly marred by inadequate pain management and infection prevention practices and by the lack of medical and psychological follow-ups. Overall, there is a "general inattention to basic human needs and privacy" (Johnson, Horga, and Fajans 2004, 190–191). In private clinics, the quality of care and accommodation is excellent, but the financial costs of abortion are high ($150 to $300 in 2021).

Since 1989, modern contraception has become available and relatively affordable. Several nongovernmental organizations (NGOs) provide partially subsidized modern contraception for all women over age 15. The insertion of intrauterine devices (IUDs) is now routinely offered by most gynecological practices. IUDs are not inexpensive, but some are more affordable than others, with prices (including the cost of the insertion procedure) ranging, in 2021, from $25 to $150. Women who opt for surgical sterilization immediately following a C-section have the procedure performed free of charge in public hospitals. However, the use of modern contraception is still limited especially among certain socioeconomic categories, despite significant changes in contraceptive education and promotion.[9] The liberalized access to safe and relatively cheap abortions has incentivized some women to avoid using modern contraception. After 1989, abortion has endured as a central method of birth control for many Romanian women (Johnson, Horga, and Fajans 2004). Once again, Oana articulated the gist of this situation: "Nowadays some [women] get abortions on their way to the workplace. It's quicker than dropping off a child to school."

The large-scale use of abortion as a method of birth control was not the only hidden reality that came to light officially in the aftermath of December 1989. When foreign journalists were granted access into the orphan shelters of the late communist era, the world discovered in horror a whole generation of neglected and malnourished children infected with human immunodeficiency virus, HIV (Kligman 1998). Meant to raise awareness about the abuses of the past, the shocking images created among Romanians unintended misunderstandings about AIDS and its transmission. The dirty, emaciated orphans were so removed from Delcel people's everyday life experiences that many women who talked to me considered themselves completely immune to HIV. The perceived radical alterity of HIV and AIDS may have been connected to some women's beliefs about not being at risk for sexually transmitted infections in general, including the human papillomavirus (HPV).

PRONATALISM RELOADED?

Despite the significant liberal shift in reproductive policies, the state has continued after 1989 to act toward disciplining its citizens' reproductive choices. A closer look at family legislation reveals how reproduction is again manipulated as part of a (this time neoliberal) social engineering project. To redress the plummeting birth rates that followed the legalization of abortion, the postcommunist governments of the last three decades have adopted new pronatalist laws (Raț 2009, 2011). The state has differentially targeted the fertility of various sociodemographic groups, incentivizing increased fertility for high income urban professionals but discouraging it for minorities—especially the Roma (Raț 2009).[10] After decades of enforced pronatalism, the new family policies have not produced the expected results. Low fertility rates are a more general European phenomenon, but Romanians' birth rates are today among the lowest in Europe (Kohler, Billari, and Ortega 2006). "Marginal" ethnic groups continue to have the highest fertility rates (Brădățan and Firebaugh 2007), triggering nationalist panic reactions about the survival of Romania, voiced at the highest political levels.

The historical trauma of Ceaușescu's pronatalism may still account for people's resistance to embrace state reproductive policies, as suggested by the public debates that followed an official abortion counseling proposal. In April 2012, a group of Liberal Party politicians initiated a proposed law mandating psychological counseling in Pregnancy Crisis Centers accredited by the Health Ministry for all women seeking an elective abortion. During counseling, pregnant women would be informed about the emotional and medical risks of terminating a pregnancy. Psychologists would describe in detail the abortion procedure, using video materials. Women would be given an ultrasound examination of the uterus that would be recorded and handed to them. Finally, counselors would explicitly state that "the embryo is a live human being from the moment of conception" and discuss with women alternatives to abortion, such as adoption, foster parents, and children shelters. After the counseling session, pregnant women would be issued a reproductive history certificate and would be granted a five-day reflection time, to reevaluate their decision to terminate the pregnancy.[11]

Political, demographic, and medical arguments overlap in the proposal.[12] Intended to grant the "right to make informed choices," the proposal conceptualizes individual women's reproduction through the lens of "the future of the entire nation." The epidemiological language of risk acquires an unexpected nationalist flavor. The document presumes that the decision to terminate a pregnancy would "negatively impact" women. In order to provide political legitimacy to their proposal, the Liberal Party deputies framed it as part of a transnational modernization project, aligned to similar abortion counseling laws from other EU countries. The deputies also invoked Romania's declining fertility rates which, they claimed, were linked to the use of abortion as a method of birth control. In 2011, it had been revealed that the total estimated number of abortions between 1958 and 2008 was more than the actual population of Romania at that moment. Most importantly, the proposal connected Romania's high incidence of breast and cervical cancers to repeated abortions, even though clinical evidence linking repeated abortions to gynecological cancers is controversial (Reeves et al. 2006; Stoicescu et al. 2017). Not unlike the pronatalist gynecological exams of the past, when women were given Pap tests to cover the real aim of detecting undeclared pregnancies, the abortion counseling proposal sought to establish its legitimacy in claiming to improve women's sexual and reproductive health. The proposal was never adopted, but the debates it generated put an end to the post-1989 "low remembrance" attitude of not openly discussing the horrors of the communist pronatalism (Anton 2009).

The debates revealed the multiplicity of voices and institutions that have an interest in regulating reproduction and reproductive health in Romania. Reactions came from "pregnancy crisis" psychologists and medical workers, gynecologists, Christian Orthodox activists, and civil society representatives. Psychologists endorsed the proposal, stressing the need for postabortion counseling as well. They had a lucrative interest in passage of the law, as the pregnancy crisis centers were to be state-sponsored. OB-GYNs expressed skepticism about the proposal's effectiveness in curbing the number of abortions. Doctors did not challenge politicians' controversial medical claims about the link between repeated abortions and gynecological cancers. Instead, OB-GYNs highlighted the practical reasons behind women's decisions to terminate unwanted pregnancies. Orthodox activists saluted the initiative, in the name of the unborn's sacred right to life. They re-semanticized the medical jargon of "risk" through a mystical reading that showed that the real risk for women was to not earn redemption after terminating a pregnancy. Civil society representatives, and especially feminist activists, expressed anger and anxiety about a proposal that, in their view, was bringing back the communist pronatalist policies and was taking away again women's reproductive autonomy. They dismissed politicians' claims that discouraging abortion would improve women's health as rhetoric and duplicitous.[13] In their view, far from exposing women to a range of informed choices, mandatory abortion counseling would drastically limit their choices. The specter of forced natality was still lurking around, threatening women to become, once again, reproductive machines to be sacrificed for the "future of the nation."

While these debates finally broke the silence that, despite free speech, had surrounded reproductive policies for more than two decades, they also had unintended consequences. The feminist critique of the proposed abortion counseling kept in the public attention the historical trauma of pronatalism, reminding older women—and presumably warning younger ones—about how untrustworthy state reproductive medicine can be. In a country report assessing abortion safety, it had been already suggested that "the historical context of abortion, especially from the Ceauşescu era, is still strong in the minds of many older Romanian women, and perhaps through oral histories, in the minds of their daughters as well" (Johnson, Horga, and Fajans 2004, 189).

I asked Oana what she thought about the proposed law to mandate abortion counseling, but surprisingly for someone so vocal, she was barely interested in this debate. Like many women of her generation, she had come of age under a materialist-atheistic ideology that equally dismissed psychology and religion. Perhaps this is why Oana was indifferent to both the arguments of the psychologists and the Orthodox associations. Like the OB-GYNs, she considered the proposal an inefficient and cynical means of discouraging women from getting abortions. Oana understood why the feminist activists referred to Ceauşescu era, but unlike them, she dismissed the possibility of an actual return to strictly enforced pronatalism. Oana was optimistic about Romania increasingly endorsing western values and granting women reproductive rights. She had reached this perspective after experiencing something that for decades had been beyond conceivable—transnational mobility.

FULSOME EUROPE, BROKEN BODIES

On New Year's Eve of 2007, as Romania was about to join the EU, hundreds of Romanian citizens lined up at the main border crossings to Hungary, eager to be the first ones to experience the long-awaited miracle of free travel. Since then, millions of Romanians have traveled abroad and have lived in EU countries.

Oana traveled to Italy, where a network of friends and neighbors from Roşiorii de Vede helped her find various unskilled jobs. Before leaving the country, Oana had inherited a house and a garden in Delcel. She planned to renovate the house with the money earned abroad. Upon her return from Italy, she moved in, alone, in 2012. Diagnosed with cervical cancer a year later, she had her uterus, cervix, fallopian tubes, and ovaries removed during a hysterectomy.

Unlike many other women from Delcel, Oana sought medical care after experiencing an extremely abundant vaginal hemorrhage. She nevertheless concedes that those who were not as active as she was in looking after their own health may still be justified: "I don't agree with women who don't go see a doctor, but I understand them. We were all scared back then." Oana implies that the repressive forms that reproductive medicine took in the past rightfully make some women avoid medical checkups in the present. Oana's own narrative of her cervical cancer surgical intervention points to some of the ways in which the historical trauma of the communist pronatalism has proliferated. In an epilogue that unexpectedly links her second clandestine abortion from decades ago to her recent hysterectomy, she recalls: "I remember it like it was yesterday, I was laying [sic] on the consultation table and that guy called the *secu*. So you may think I am not sane . . ."—Oana looks at me intently as she pauses for a moment—". . . when I had to lay down again on my back on that [surgical] table right before the [hysterectomy] surgery, I felt that man's presence in the room."

Oana's confession reveals the mechanisms of traumatic memory in action. Unlike ordinary memory, which is social, traumatic memory keeps the consciousness captive "in an ever-renewing present of existential horror" (van der Kolk 2014, 179, see also 182). One of the Romanian women interviewed by Kligman (1998, 185) kept associating the image of a chair with the feeling of humiliation, after experiencing an embarrassing heavy hemorrhage while seated in a chair in her office, hours after an attempted back-alley abortion. Similarly, Oana has a disturbing flashback of her second clandestine abortion at the very moment when she is about to receive a potentially life-saving surgery. The memory of trauma is so powerful and so deeply inscribed in the body that it overtakes for a moment the fear of cancer, of suffering, of dying. Furthermore, it is through a hauntology lexicon that Oana articulates her brief moment of hesitancy about the cervical cancer intervention. The abuses of the former regime seem to haunt Oana, who literally sees the ghost that connects gynecological procedures with political surveillance. The memory of trauma is "tied to the body" and rendered manifest through somatization (van der Kolk 2014; Brison 1999), but it is also tied to a place as well. Oana experiencing the spectral apparition in the surgery room highlights the multilayered phenomenological temporalities of care. As I show in more detail in chapter 5, the "repetitions that connect different social, political, sectarian, and ontological orders" can make hospitals sites of "uncanny and otherworldly presences" (Varley and Varma 2018, 630). Oana's life unfolds like a Greek tragedy, from the prologue of the first underground abortion to the catharsis of the final hysterectomy. From this closing vantage point, Oana contemplates the paradoxes of her reproductive life:

> My friend and I were only twenty-four, but both of us wished we were older, much older, so that we would not bear children anymore ... and now [after the hysterectomy], I feel mutilated and I wish I were younger and healthier.

CONCLUSIONS

Oana's and her peers' reproductive experiences of the past continue to shape their responses to sexual and reproductive care. The 1948 criminalization of abortion had already created an incipient market for clandestine pregnancy terminations, but it was the 1966 decree that boosted the back-alley abortion industry in the 1970s and 1980s. The pronatalist regime restricted women's reproductive rights and limited their access to crucial medical care. This prompted women to challenge the state as a reliable and resourceful provider of reproductive care. Resistance to state reproductive medicine took the form of engaging in informal and personalized tactics aimed at securing access to means of fertility control. The ability to clandestinely navigate alternative networks of resources and connections was crucial to women's desires to manage unwanted fertility (Kligman 1998; Miroiu and Dragomir 2010). The system affected everybody, even those who keenly desired to reproduce.

Although the communist pronatalist policies were discontinued in 1989, three decades later, they still haunt private lives and public narratives. The precedents set by past reproductive policies were invoked to fuel debates over abortion counseling. For those who experienced the political surveillance of reproduction as traumatic, state medicine appeared as irrelevant and ineffective. The memory of past reproductive injustice deters some women from engaging with state-driven reproductive care that also includes cervical cancer prevention, as I show in more detail especially in chapters 3, 4 and 6 (see also Andreassen et al. 2017). While not all women have traumatic recollections of past reproductive events, many are ambivalent about state reproductive medicine.

Romanian women's experiences of navigating the reproductive landscapes of the communist era have produced enduring effects that, decades later, still impact their views on sexual and reproductive health and health care. However, women were not the only ones subjected to traumatic family and reproductive policies. Pronatalism impacted men, too, although in different ways than it affected women. As I demonstrate in the next chapter, in order to better understand the most intimate and enduring effects that past reproductive policies have had on Romanian women, we need to also locate Romanian men within the realm of reproduction.

2 · REPRODUCTIVE INVISIBILITY

> After they moved out from the bed, after they had sex, the men disappeared.
> I never saw the men around, during the abortions, during the delivery,
> during the time women had gynecological problems. I didn't see the men
> too much. I don't know where they were. (Iepan 2005)

This is how Adrian Sângerozan, a male OB-GYN who practiced medicine during the pronatalist years, sums up his encounters—or rather the lack thereof—with his patients' male relatives. Coming from a professional who recalls the inner workings of reproductive policies intended to force women into pregnancy and childbirth, Doctor Sângerozan's interest in men's whereabouts is surprising. In traditional patriarchal contexts of gender segregation—such as those of pre–World War II rural and peri-urban Romania—it was customary for men to stay away from reproductive events such as births, miscarriages, and abortions. However, men have continued to stay invisible to women's reproduction, even during the allegedly gender-egalitarian regime of the communists and long after the communism's demise. Men's invisibility has had important consequences for women's reproductive health and well-being.

In this chapter, I examine the presumed reproductive invisibility of Romanian men during and after communism. Following Sângerozan's observation, I locate men within the historical, political and cultural contexts of reproduction in communist and postcommunist Romania. I consider the shifting ways in which patriarchal values and practices have shaped both women's and men's ideas about reproductive health and health care, including access to cervical cancer prevention.

In situating men in relation to the "structures of feeling" (Williams and Orrom 1954) of reproduction, I build on several theoretical contributions of anthropology. First, following anthropologists who reconsider men's participation in human reproduction (Inhorn 2012; Gutmann 2011; Wentzell 2013), I reinsert men into the realm of reproduction. Romanian men's lives were also shaped by the communist pronatalist policies, even if in less conspicuous ways, and acknowledging this can deepen our understanding of the reproductive challenges that both women and men faced. Second, I integrate suggestions from colonial and postcolonial studies

(White 2000; Chapman 2010) and from the anthropology of language as performance (Kligman 1988; Besnier 2009), to consider human interactions through the lens of the more inclusive category of "agency" rather than as a dynamic of power-versus-resistance. Power and resistance cannot always account for the shifting nature of lived reality (Foucault 1982; Butler 1997; Ortner 1995). As I show in this chapter, men managed to preserve patriarchal privileges within their families even when subjected to forms of citizenship emasculation by a totalitarian state. Thus, men were simultaneously powerless and powerful. Their everyday lives consisted of shifting back and forth between these two conditions. The notion of "agency"—understood as historically and culturally embedded intentionality (Besnier 2009)—can help us grasp the fluctuating nature of men's reproductive roles during and after communism.

To Doctor Sângerozan and other OB-GYNs who practiced in the 1970s and 1980s, men were oddly absent from the bedside of their female partners and relatives (Iepan 2005). As I demonstrate in this chapter, men are in fact inconspicuously present in reproductive contexts in multiple places, playing various and sometimes contradictory roles. Their image is contingent on the discourses through which they are construed. Drawing from a mix of primary and secondary sources, I look for men in ideological discourses and in everyday practices by comparing state propaganda about gender equality to recent ethnographic observations of interactions between men and women. Next, I locate men in women's private accounts, before also considering the claims that men themselves make or fail to make about their own participation to reproduction. All these sources converge in revealing another set of systemic contingencies that may illuminate the current cervical cancer crisis—the persistence of patriarchal relations in contemporary Romania. This is a consequential fact when promoting sexual and reproductive health care for women, as shown in the design and the implementation of the 2008–2020 HPV vaccination campaigns. I examine cervical cancer prevention advertising, showing how it was tacitly informed by the notion that men and boys have nothing to do with women's and girls' reproductive health. I conclude noting that filmmaking and journalism are the few unlikely places from which men have been either denouncing past reproductive policies or expressing nationalist-flavored nostalgia for pronatalism.

"LIFE COMRADES" . . . OR NOT?

The communist regime challenged traditional patriarchy[1] and recast women as men's "life comrades." Massive rural to urban migration and industrialization produced a demographic shift that transformed previous residential arrangements of new wives moving in with their husbands' relatives (patrilocality) to the newlyweds living on their own in the cities (neolocality).[2] By the mid-1970s and especially during the "Golden Age" of the 1980s, images of Nicolae

Ceaușescu and of his wife Elena—the ultimate life comrades—were displayed everywhere in public places. Whether in allegoric or realistic portrayals, the couple was depicted, often oversized, side by side, embodying the ideal comradeship between husband and wife (Buchel and Carmine 2008). Communist etiquette also required the gender-neutral "comrade" (*tovarăș/tovarășă*) as the term of address and reference in all public interactions, replacing the previous use of "mister," "missus," "sir," and "madam"—considered "bourgeois" and obsolete (Ghodsee 2011).

Traditional patriarchal values continued to inform state propaganda under communism. Despite the regime's claims of having secured gender equality, women's and men's public and domestic roles were uneven (Miroiu 2010; Jinga 2015). Under communism, women were overwhelmed by the triple burden of double workdays—that is, the expectation that they would shift daily between their responsibilities as mothers and wives, housekeepers and cooks, and career workers (Kligman 1998; Du Plessix Gray 1989; Miroiu 2010). Although men, as communist citizens, were politically disempowered by a totalitarian paternalist state, they preserved patriarchal prerogatives within their own families. Under the communist dictatorship, the family became the last patriarchal stronghold to men otherwise emasculated by the repressive state (Miroiu 2010). As we shall see in the next section, throughout the communist regime and after, domestic violence against women was high. While men's subordination to the state was only public, women's was both public and private.

The vision behind the criminalization of abortion in 1966 was also a patriarchal one. According to Decree 770, abortion was legal only for women over age 45 or for those who already had four and later five living children. Other exceptions that allowed an abortion were endangerment of a woman's life, proof that the woman was physically or psychologically debilitated, the congenital malformation of the fetus, or a pregnancy that was the result of incest or rape. These exceptions to the law reflected its patriarchal character, since men were held accountable for their own sexual behavior only in extreme cases such as rape and incest (Kligman 1998, 249). By reinforcing the patriarchal stereotypes of husbands' sexual prerogatives, the pronatalist policies made marital intimacy a locus of struggle for both women and men. Furthermore, public transcripts of the two executive meetings of the Central Committee of the Romanian Communist Party, from August 2 to September 27, 1966, held in preparation of the new abortion legislation, reveal that the proposed law to criminalize abortion was debated exclusively by the party's male leaders. They assumed the role of reproductive policy makers on behalf of women and crafted self-serving policies that exonerated them of reproductive accountability for their sexuality. Voicing traditional patriarchal views, Ceaușescu had the final say, enforcing his vision of a motherhood disconnected from the lived realities of sexuality and modern contraception (Doboș, Jinga, and Soare 2010). Significantly, in December 1989, it was also a majority of men—the political leaders emerging following the ousting of Ceaușescu—who abrogated Decree 770.[3]

The post-decree baby boom of 1967 to 1968 brought Romania to 20 million people in 1969. To mark the historical demographic milestone, the Communist Party organized an official event during which a young mother ceremoniously presented to the supreme leader Ceaușescu a three-month old baby boy—the 20 millionth Romanian citizen (Kligman 1998; Iepan 2005). Presumably, the baby had been chosen randomly from the 1,000 newborns of June 20, 1969, using a computing machine from the National Institute of Statistics. The 20 millionth Romanian celebration shows that the pronatalist propaganda capitalized on both traditional and state patriarchy. Although "arbitrarily" selected, the 20 millionth citizen proved to have "the ideal" gender, ethnic, and class profile. The baby was a boy born to recently urbanized working-class parents of pure Romanian ethnic origins (Iepan 2005). Whereas the new ideal man was supposedly engaged in a lifelong comradeship with his female counterpart, the quintessential communist citizen remained a male.

"MOTHER-IN-LAW, SOUR HAW..."

Before communism, in predominantly rural Romania, when wives moved in with their husbands' relatives they became, as daughters-in-law, assimilated into their new families. A mother-in-law would closely monitor her daughter-in-law's conduct, including reproductive events such as miscarriages or births (Voland and Beise 2005). After giving birth to sons, a wife would eventually become an authoritative figure herself, closely watching, as a mother-in-law, the initiation and reproductive conduct of the next generation of daughters-in-law.

Traditional patriarchy persisted under communism and resurfaced again after 1989, sometimes in forms reminiscent of pre-WWII Romania. Reverse urban to rural migration produced a shift back to patrilocal residence in some rural and peri-urban areas, like Delcel. With the postcommunist restructuring of the economy and the closing of urban factories, some of the recently urbanized working-class families returned to the countryside to live with their older relatives who had been left behind. For those who stayed in the cities, reemerging patrilocal living arrangements were often the result of pauperization.[4] Domestic violence against women and marital rape, although legally prohibited, was and is still often considered a husband's prerogative (Rujoiu 2011).

As I show in the following vignettes, in Roșiorii de Vede, traditional patriarchy has never become completely obsolete. Traditional patrilineal rules of descent[5] seem to be enduring, along with the gendered division of labor within the household, the valuing of wives for their reproductive contribution to the lineage, and a general preference for sons over daughters expressed by both women and men.[6] More significantly, patriarchal attitudes and practices still shape the sexual and reproductive health of women from Delcel. Ethnographic observation allows us to document current forms of patriarchy in Romania while showcasing the diversity of women's actual responses to patriarchal pressures.

Except for her tired, sunburned hands, Ileana does not show her age. At fifty-nine, her short hair is dyed a dark-blond shade; her face is almost wrinkle-free. After completing ten years of school more than forty years ago, Ileana married at age 19. Like the majority of married women from Delcel, she moved in with her in-laws. She recalls with resigned sadness the first major incident with her new relatives. Sometime in the late 1970s, her older son, then age 5, had beaten up a classmate, and the teacher sent Ileana a written note asking her to come to school to discuss the incident. Ileana had been busy all day, cleaning and cooking in preparation for the upcoming blessing of the house—an Eastern Orthodox ritual held to consecrate new or recently renovated construction. Upon seeing the teacher's note, Ileana's mother-in-law decided that *she* would go to school and talk to the teacher. Ileana reminded her that the teacher had specifically asked to talk to the mother—not the grandmother. Deeply offended, the mother-in-law reported the disobedience to her son—Ileana's husband—who immediately settled the dispute by beating Ileana. After seizing the festive dishes that Ileana had prepared, Ileana's husband and her mother-in-law left together to moaşa's place, celebrating there and leaving a sorrowful Ileana alone at home. In this region of southern Romania, the husband's older sister is called moaşa—a term used to refer to a midwife, literally meaning "the old man's wife." Before the 1950s medicalization of births, a moaşa used to cut the umbilical cord of her younger brother's newborns, acting like a real midwife. Since then, she has played only a symbolic role as an initiator during rites of passage associated with a newborn's first days. What made this early marriage episode particularly painful to Ileana was the realization that, although both her mother-in-law and her sister-in-law had once been young daughters-in-law in their own households, they showed no compassion toward Ileana.

Ileana's story illustrates one of the most striking features of traditional patriarchy: Assimilation of new wives into the husband's family is marked by women's antagonism. Kinship cohesion outperforms gender solidarity (Stone 2006). In Romania, there are numerous ethnographic accounts (Florea Marian [1892] 2009) and folkloric tales about the tense relationships between mothers and their daughters-in-law. In one of the most popular examples, a folktale by Ion Creangă ([1875] 1978), three daughters-in-law end up killing their abusive mother-in-law while singing together:

Mother-in-law, sour haw,
Ripe all day in the sun
Sweeter sure you'll get none

Ripe all autumn thereupon
You're still sour as a lemon.[7]

The mother-in-law's monologue at the beginning of the story provides a glimpse into how she guards and reproduces patriarchal customs:

> I'll keep a strict eye on the daughters-in-law, I'll make them work, and keep a tight rein on them, not letting them outdoors when my sons are away. That's how my mother-in-law, may God rest her in peace, behaved toward me. And my husband, may God forgive him, could not complain I deceived him or squandered things . . . although at times he did suspect me and kicked me some. . . .[8]

After Ileana's mother-in-law died, family relations remained strained because of *moaşa*'s repeated interferences into Ileana's life. Ileana is now herself a mother-in-law and a grandmother. Her two adult sons work and live with their families in Bucharest. One day, during my stay in Delcel, one of the sons, Claudiu, came to visit his parents with his wife and children. For the occasion, *moaşa* was also invited to join them. She arrived with her own adult daughter, bringing presents and sweet treats for Ileana's grandchildren. When *moaşa* offered the candies to the youngsters, Claudiu politely declined her gift, explaining to her that the children were not allowed to have sweets before lunch. Ignoring their father's intervention, *moaşa* continued to offer the treats to the children. Eventually, Claudiu bluntly reminded *moaşa* that his children were not under her authority. Deeply offended, *moaşa* withdrew, not before making a comment about "these modern times when young people no longer obey their elders." As the older living woman of the lineage, *moaşa* assumed that she had authority over the entire family, including Ileana's grandchildren. During our conversations, Ileana's attitude was one of resigned compliance. By now, she was used to be repeatedly humiliated by her female in-laws. However, Ileana confessed to me that after that painful event from her early marriage years, she made a promise to herself that, regardless of circumstances and custom, she would be nice to her own future daughters-in-law. Indeed, Ileana's interactions with her daughters-in-law were remarkably affable. Her behavior was the result of a conscious, deliberate choice. Ileana's willingness to break with the patriarchal tradition of the "sour mother-in-law"—while easier to carry on because of her sons' neolocal residence—is remarkable, as it represents an active, engaged response to forms of patriarchal oppression.

About three months after I settled in Delcel, as we chatted one morning over a cup of Turkish coffee, Ileana told me about her seventy-four-year-old knowledgeable neighbor, Maria. From Ileana's description of Maria, I could already imagine a possible key study participant. With my curiosity sparked, that same afternoon I went with Ileana to Maria's place. We stopped in front of an iron fence. A handwritten cardboard sign that read *Butelii 12,5 kg 40 lei* ("Propane tanks 12.5 kilograms 40 lei") was attached to the gate with a piece of bent wire, indicating that the host was an entrepreneur who, for a fee, traded empty propane tanks for refilled ones. Ileana knew that Maria's dog was on a leash in the backyard, so she just yelled out hello to Maria while we let ourselves into the courtyard. We took a narrow concrete alley crossing the most beautiful flower and vegetable garden I had seen in the whole neighborhood. At the end of the alley was a small, whitewashed house. A shrunken, wrinkled, sunburned woman with a lively and commanding presence greeted us at the front door. Maria kept her head covered in the old-fashioned way, with a floral kerchief tied at the back of her neck. We entered the parlor, leaving our shoes on the threshold. Our host invited Ileana and me to sit and poured soda into ceramic mugs. Throughout my stay in Delcel, Maria would become one the most outspoken study participant, who would often force me outside of my comfort zone of scripted questionnaires with her inquisitive and humorous comments. During this first visit at her house I felt intimidated by her curious, intelligent gaze. Born to illiterate farmers, Maria is one of ten surviving siblings. She attended only two years of school before withdrawing to help her parents with farming work. After having been married for twelve years to a violent alcoholic husband, she divorced him. She told me that, two years before my arrival in Delcel, she was feeling unwell. Fearing a tuberculosis (TB) diagnosis, her family doctor sent her to the local hospital's imaging laboratory for a chest X-ray. The film showed a suspicious spot on her lung. Alarmed, one of her sons took Maria to a specialist in Bucharest. On a closer examination, the suspected TB mark on her lung turned out to be the scar of a rib broken during an episode of domestic violence years ago. Maria earned the sole custody of their two young children. She showed me several gold-plastic-framed family pictures of her two now-adult sons who had recently migrated to Spain with their families. During our subsequent conversations, Maria would always brag about her efforts to raise them as a single mother.

Whereas Maria proudly assumed motherhood, she also recalled the fights with her ex-mother-in-law who often interfered with Maria's reproductive choices: "I have two [children], only two, but my mother-in-law used to tell me *you must have five children. . . .* My mother-in-law kept repeating *have another one, have another one, have another one.*" Maria resisted the reproductive pressures of a mother-in-law who urged her to contribute to the lineage, and an alcoholic husband who forced her into nonconsensual sexual relations, by having abortions. In the absence of any form of contraception—natural, traditional, or modern— she alleged that she had thirty abortions during her marriage, both before and after 1966. Repeated abortions became her way to challenge everyday patriarchy. Compared to Ileana and some other peers, Maria was atypically bold, as proven by her decision to leave her husband and assume the status of a single mother in a community where divorced women were twice stigmatized—for breaking with traditional family model and for defying the communist legislation designed to curb divorce rates. While Maria's disturbing history of domestic violence, marital rape, and repeated abortions took place in the 1960s, as recently as 2002 there was still no legislation against family violence and marital rape (Roman 2003). In the name of conjugal rights, women have been subjected to forms of domestic violence ranging from verbal abuse to beating and rape. In 2003 and 2004, caving in to international pressure, the parliament promulgated laws prohibiting domestic violence and redefining rape to include sexual assault by family members (Rujoiu 2011). However, marital rapes continue to be underreported because of the belief—sometimes shared by both men and women—that domestic intimate violence is not a form of abuse (Rujoiu 2011). Domestic violence, such as inflicted on Ileana and Maria, and the marital rape to which Maria was subjected are linked to patriarchal reproductive pressures on women, which, in turn, impact their sexual and reproductive health and well-being. Enabled by their own mothers as mothers-in-law, in the name of patriarchal reproductive imperatives, men are absolved of the consequences of their (sometimes violent) sexuality.

A FEW GOOD MEN, MANY BAD MEN, AND NO GRAY MEN

To locate Romanian men in the realm of reproduction, I have juxtaposed propagandistic accounts from before 1989 to ethnographic data gathered between 2005 and 2013 in Roşiorii de Vede. In this section, I consider women's explicit opinions about men's presumed reproductive invisibility. I integrate findings from other ethnographies, such as Florin Iepan's documentary *Children of the Decree* (2005), which features several women's abortion stories from 1966 to 1989, and Gail Kligman's book *The Politics of Duplicity* (1998, ch. 6), which reproduces "bitter memories" of the clandestine abortion accounts of women and obstetricians. Mihaela Miroiu and Otilia Dragomir (2010) edited a collection of birthing stories told by twenty women who gave birth in Romania before and after 1989. Other ethnologists and anthropologists occasionally cite women's abortion or birthing accounts (Anton 2009, 2014; Bărbulescu 1998). I also use fictional and anecdotal references that can provide a particular depth to women's accounts about men's (lack of) involvement with reproduction. First, I consider references from the 2007 fictional movie *4 Months, 3 Weeks and 2 Days*, by director Cristian Mungiu, which tells the anticlimactic story of a back-alley abortion gone wrong in 1980s Romania. Mungiu explores the desperation and cynicism that shaped power relations on the market of clandestine abortions, as pregnant Găbiţa and her best friend Otilia face Mister Bebe, the abortionist. Despite being awarded the Golden Palm at the Cannes Film Festival, *4 Months, 3 Weeks and 2 Days* had a rather cold reception in Romania. Several women from Delcel told me that, on learning about the movie's topic, they decided against watching it because they didn't want to see their reproductive traumas commodified on the big screen. Although fictional, the story the film tells is plausible, and its *cinéma-vérité* quality makes Mungiu's movie a credible source to locate men in women's reproductive accounts. Second, I draw on overheard and only half-understood stories about illegal abortions—whispers, unfinished sentences, rumors, and gossip that surrounded me during my teen years in the late 1980s and whose full meanings I grasped later in my adult life. While ethnographic, fictional, and anecdotal accounts are, each in their own way, partial and subjective, they are valuable when corroborated with documentary sources, because they fill the gaps that exist in official discourses.

In the light of these sources, let us revisit Oana's abortion diaries from chapter 1. As stated there, Oana had two clandestine abortions that she secured by activating networks of connections, acquaintances, and even strangers. She then attempted to frame her abortions as miscarriages. To highlight that these networks of informal connections are gendered, I edited this time the English translation of Oana's words, by adding the gender of nouns:[9]

It happened sometimes in '75 or '76. My mom had this acquaintance—a [female] pharmacist—and she provided me with a full battery of injections. . . . And I took [the injections] and then I waited and waited and eventually I started to bleed and I had a huge hemorrhage. I called the ambulance. . . . The [male] doctor asked me what had happened. I lied that we had moved, and I had carried heavy furniture. . . . At the hospital they gave me a vacuum aspiration and let me go without further questioning.

The second time was worse. There were more restrictions. Many [male] obstetricians and women had been jailed for illegal abortions. . . . I took those injections again, but nothing happened, time passed, nothing [happened]. Then, a [female] friend of my sister-in-law referred me to a [male] doctor who was just part-time affiliated with the maternity hospital. I went to the ambulatory room of the hospital, the [male] doctor tried something, but with no result. A few days later, a [female] relative of my sister-in-law's [female] friend arranged things with a [female] medical nurse. . . . So I went to my sister-in-law's relative's place, at her home, and there the nurse inserted a catheter. . . .

I ran to the hospital . . . and then the [male] doctor came in and I showed him the bleeding. Of course, again, *What did you do? When was the last menstruation?* He noticed the blood clots and scheduled me for a vacuum aspiration.

Finally, I was brought into the surgery room, I [was] laid on the table and there was a man right there, not a doctor, a [male] civilian. He called *secu* [Securitate, the secret police]. *We have here a patient, heavily bleeding, with clots, we believe that the embryo is compromised. We cannot keep her pregnancy, so we ask permission to give her a vacuum aspiration.* Only after *secu* agreed, they proceeded with the aspiration.

During a follow-up discussion, Oana added the following to her abortion recollections: "My husband didn't want to hear about condoms. I had gotten some
from my mom's [female] friend, the pharmacist. Later, I heard that there were
[male] doctors who clandestinely inserted diaphragms."

The informal networks that Oana activated to secure an abortion are gendered. Female solidarity is particularly remarkable, occasionally making translation difficult, as personal connections and relationships unfold in a string of
genitive cases, such as "a [female] relative of my sister-in-law's [female] friend."
In Oana's account, as well as in some other women's stories, men are not invisible. They are instead found in multiple and unstable roles that shift back and
forth between powerful and powerless.

One of the roles in which men are cast in women's accounts is that of the
husband/male partner. Unwilling to co-participate to contraception,[10] the husband is often absent from the clandestine abortion networks. Some women confessed to blaming and hating their own husbands for exerting their "conjugal
rights" without considering the potential reproductive consequences.[11] Doctor
Onicescu, another male obstetrician featured in Iepan's documentary, underscored the disconnect between men's sexuality and reproduction: "Men wanted
to have sex. Men wanted women to avoid having too many children, but they
didn't want to have anything to do with the police, the prosecutors. . . . In other
words: *you deal with it*" (Iepan 2005).

Some women categorized men based on their reproductive solidarity with
their female partners as either "good men" or "bad men." "I don't know of
any gray men," asserted former national TV presenter Delia Budeanu, using the
color metaphor to convey the polarization of men's support to women, when
interviewed by Iepan (2005). Irina, a fifty-eight-year-old woman from Delcel,
told me how atypical her husband was. A "good man," he played a crucial role in
arranging a safe clandestine abortion for her. He declined the services of an
available back-alley abortion provider who had no formal medical training and
struggled, using his connections, to find a medical nurse willing to perform the
procedure surreptitiously at her house. However, during subsequent abortions,
Irina's husband did not get involved anymore. Significantly, in Mungiu's movie,
there is not even a veiled allusion to the male sexual partner who helped conceive the fetus. Women's deaths from complications of clandestine abortions
provoked surprise and shock in oblivious husbands (Iepan 2005), whose invisibility sometimes continued into their deceased wives' remembrance rituals.[12]
Under pronatalism, husbands' lack of involvement with their wives' reproductive experiences was to many women an additional source of stress.

Some of the men to whom women refer in their accounts are OB-GYNs. They
also are typologically polarized and cast as either the "good doctor"—who performs illegal abortions and inserts diaphragms bought on the black market, bravely
defying political surveillance and risking jail time—or the "bad doctor"—who

acts like an agent of oppression, performs mandatory gynecological controls at women's workplaces, and mercilessly questions patients who present with heavy bleeding (Bărbulescu 1998; Doboş, Jinga, and Soare 2010). However, on a closer look, it becomes evident that, rather than either resisting or complying with the biopolitics of reproduction, doctors used their agency as system's insiders in more nuanced ways. The doctor interrogates Oana the first time she pretends to have a miscarriage, but he then gives her a vacuum aspiration and discharges her without further reporting. This cannot be replicated a second time, when the doctor himself is under the civilian's surveillance during the medical exam. Some doctors deliberately occupy interstitial public-private spaces that allow them to display a certain degree of agency. I noted in chapter 1 the liminality of the "part-time affiliated" doctor who becomes available only when contacted through informal communication channels, but then attempts to interrupt Oana's pregnancy inside the public hospital. Other male OB-GYNs—like those featured in Iepan's documentary—craft a genderless professional voice for themselves, which allows them to comfortably denounce the lack of reproductive accountability of their patients' husbands, without having to acknowledge their own manhood. During pronatalism, some male OB-GYNs occupy fluid spaces and relationships, from where they can navigate the paradoxes of being involved with and detached from the horrors of the political control over women's reproduction.

In some real-life cases, as well as in fiction, the abortionist is a man.[13] Mungiu's movie prominently features "Mister Bebe"—a back-alley abortion provider apparently lacking formal medical training. Yet, even this character carries a great deal of ambiguity, as he is both a savior and a perpetrator. As a skilled abortion provider, he succeeds in helping Găbiţa get rid of her unwanted pregnancy, but as a man, he asks for sexual favors in exchange of his abortion services. Mister Bebe's lack of concern for the reproductive consequences of his sexuality reinscribes the cycle of forced reproduction that he helps break.

One of the most enigmatic male figures in women's accounts is "the civilian." He is usually the man in charge of the actual enforcement of political control over female reproduction. Women's stories feature various men playing this role. Sometimes the civilian can be a prosecutor, other times he is a political activist or even the foreman, as in this former textile factory female worker's recollection of the way she and her workmates were summoned for mandatory controls: "The foreman would come next to the weaving looms and say: *You have to go to the consultation room*" (Iepan 2005).

Finally, the secret police or the regular police representative is always a man—whom the popular culture under communism sarcastically represented as a stereotypical blue-eyed character, wearing a leather jacket. He is the one responsible with issuing the final decision regarding suspicious reproductive events. This man's physical presence is hidden. In Oana's account, he exists only as a voice at the other end of the telephone call. Yet, it is precisely the ubiquity of his invisibility that makes him such a powerful reproductive player.

In conclusion, when men are not absent from women's reproduction narratives, the roles they play are fluid, difficult to grasp and to categorize into neat typologies. Rather than conceptualizing men as invisible, women's stories draw attention to the shifting quality of men's agency within the realm of reproduction. Men themselves are almost always voiceless in women's accounts. We are left wondering about men's own claims about their reproductive contribution. Therefore, let us give men the floor.

A MAN'S WORK: PLAYING WITH THE BABY

In contrast to the relative abundance of archival and ethnographic sources that situate men in official discourses and in women's private accounts, the evidence to document men's own claims about their reproductive roles is scarce. As a young woman doing fieldwork in a peri-urban location of southern Romania, my interactions with men were bound to local stereotypes about gender roles. Because of my gender, age, education, marital status, and reproductive condition, the men from Delcel resisted my attempts to initiate semiformal interviews. The occasional informal conversations with men would often end prematurely, with them dismissing my questions as "female stuff" (*treburi femeieşti*). Given these circumstances, I used a survey to learn about the claims that men themselves made or failed to make about their participation to reproduction.

Adapting a survey that Kideckel (1993) conducted in the Ţara Oltului region of Romania, I listed forty-three household chores or routine activities/tasks. For each chore, twenty-five women and twenty-one men indicated the gender of the person expected to perform it, using a five-grade scale: only women, especially women, both women and men, especially men, only men. Even though they completed the survey separately, for most of the household chores both women and men agreed about the descriptor from the scale when they indicated the gender corresponding to each activity. Table 3 illustrates the gendered distribution of labor in households.

Table 4 illustrates women's and men's disagreement about the gender distribution of some household chores, which I call "disputed" chores. They are disputed in theory, since women and men used different descriptors from the scale to designate who was responsible for these activities. The chores are also disputed in action since, according to my observations, overlapping occurs.

As shown in these tables, childcare is seen by both women and men as an almost exclusively female activity. The survey, follow-up discussions, and ethnographic observations revealed that fathers' involvement in childcare varied from one household to the next, ranging from quasi-total neglect to punctual but

TABLE 3.   Gender division of labor in Delcel community, Roșiorii de Vede, Teleorman County, Romania.

Only or Especially Women	Both Women and Men	Only or Especially Men
Feeding the baby/children	Contributing to the household budget	Cutting wood
Bathing the baby/children	Strolling the baby	Feeding the animals
Dressing the baby/children	Shopping	Cleaning the stables
Preparing meals	Buying and carrying propane tanks	Mowing
Cooking	Digging the garden	Beekeeping
Washing dishes	Watering the garden	Raising pigeons
Baking bread	Weeding	Cutting trees
Painting Easter eggs	Sweeping the courtyard	Pruning grapevines
Sorting laundry		Fixing fences
Laundry		Plowing
Rinsing clothing		Harrowing
Hanging laundry to dry		
Wrapping clothing		
Ironing		
Sweeping		
Carrying water		
Collecting eggs from domestic birds		

TABLE 4.   Gender division of labor in Delcel community, Roșiorii de Vede, Teleorman County, Romania. Disputed chores.

Activity/Chore	Women's Opinion about Who Is in Charge	Men's Opinion about Who Is in Charge
Organizing the household work	Especially women	Both women and men
Playing with the baby/children	Both women and men	Especially men
Vacuum cleaning	Only women	Both women and men
Dusting	Only women	Both women and men
Cleaning carpets	Especially women	Both women and men
Gathering wood	Especially men	Both women and men
Whitewashing the trees	Both women and men	Only men

consistent chores, such as feeding a baby with a bottle, taking a baby out for a stroll, or playing with the baby. Fathers seemed to be less interested in caring for girls, especially when they were not the first born. Out of thirty-three mothers, twenty confessed during our conversations that their husbands were at some point uninterested in taking care of their baby girls. Overall, fathers and men do not participate in childcare. When they do, their contribution is usually more symbolic than practical. Both women and men agreed about all aspects of childcare (feeding, bathing, dressing, and strolling) being only or especially women's work, except for "playing with the baby/children"; this activity is a disputed chore. While women admitted that men were also involved in the rather amusing, pleasant, and easy chore of playing with the baby, men tried to appropriate this activity by classifying it as "especially men." Ana, a twenty-nine-year-old housewife, reflects on fathers' (lack of) involvement in childcare: "It depends. If he loves the baby, he will come and watch when the baby takes a bath. Or, when the baby cries while the mother sleeps, he sometimes goes and comforts the baby."

Ana perceives paternal love as conditional ("If he loves the baby"). Also, she situates a father's care into a contemplative rather than practical ground ("he will come and watch when the baby takes a bath"). Ana's observation aligns with both women's and men's ideas about men being involved in "playing with the baby," but not in feeding, bathing, or dressing the baby. This distribution of childcare chores reveals that the expectations that both women and men have for themselves and for their partners in terms of rearing roles are gender specific. During my stay in Delcel, I seldom witnessed husbands and wives or men and women sharing the same chore. Even on those rare occasions when I observed couples working together, it was more a contingent decision than a customary occurrence (figure 5). Unloading a wagon of logs or sorting the body parts

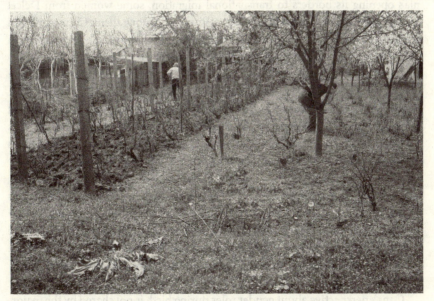

FIGURE 5. Husband and wife from Delcel working the garden "together." The woman (left) does the strenuous work of digging the garden while the man is pruning the grapevines. (Photo by the author.)

of a freshly slaughtered pig were time-sensitive actions that required the joint involvement of men and women. Virtually all chores, including those they claimed to be gender neutral (see table 3), were carried out by men and women separately or alternatively, but not together. With respect to labor in general and childcare in particular, women and men belong to highly segregated social worlds in rural and peri-urban southern Romania.

The medicalization of birth did not challenge traditional gender roles that assign men the privilege of nonparticipation. Today, most men from Delcel consider birth exclusively a female activity, and they are reluctant to even consider being present in the birthing room. Similarly, most women neither expect nor want their husbands to be present at a child's birth. When I asked them about their husbands' whereabouts during delivery, women told me that while they were giving birth, the men were in the maternity hospital hallway, in a nearby bar, or at home either smoking, drinking coffee or alcohol, or praying. Most of Romania's public maternity hospitals have policies that do not allow family members to attend birth. During an informal discussion, Gabriela's thirty-eight-year-old husband told me that, although he had been granted exceptional access into the birthing room to be with his wife (owing to his personal connections with the medical personnel from Polizu Maternity Hospital in Bucharest), he declined to participate because birth "was not something to be seen by a man."

Prompted by an increased awareness of less patriarchal alternatives to gender roles in western European countries that they witnessed in the aftermath of Romania's opening its borders to transnational migration, some women from Delcel voiced their aspiration to challenge the status quo. Among them, Oana expressed the most cosmopolitan views about gender roles. She elaborated her arguments in a progress-oriented, modernist frame, unintentionally reproducing feminist statements. When I elicited her advice to an expectant mother, Oana promptly retorted: "Work out during pregnancy and, if you can afford to, have a water delivery. That would be modern. And invite the baby's father into the delivery room. He will respect you more...." She paused for a moment, only to add, with a laugh, "Unless he faints before [you deliver]." I asked her to elaborate on the reasons fathers should attend birth. Oana passionately explained:

> To learn to respect the woman more. To realize that birth is female work and is beautiful after all. And to see how it really takes place. They conceived the baby together. He should see how it works, and he should participate and see how the birth takes place. I would have liked to have [my husband] with me. I would have felt better. But this is embarrassing for some. Not many women would accept it.

Oana's perspective about gender roles during birth is not shared by the majority of women in Delcel. Yet it is important to acknowledge this incipient plurality of opinions. Also, in large urban areas, gender roles have shifted toward a less segregated paradigm of reproduction. In private clinics, fathers are encouraged to attend birth. In recent years, it has become common for men to accompany women at prenatal medical visits. However, men are not present in the consultation room during the pelvic exam. They are invited by the OB-GYN to join their female partners only for the ultrasound scan, which is the most entertaining part of the exam. The parents-to-be watch together images of their future child projected on a computer screen. Fathers' involvement with reproductive issues is, again, more contemplative than practical.

INVISIBLE MEN, INVISIBLE BOYS

Even though men's patriarchal elusiveness from all matters of reproduction has proved to be largely a cultural and political construct, it has had, nevertheless, concrete consequences on women's reproductive health and well-being. Unlike other countries, Romania did not include men as decision-makers in their children's health or boys in the target group for receiving the human papillomavirus (HPV) vaccine. In the United States, HPV vaccine advertising has shifted the focus from girls and women solely to include boys and men. The 2006 "One less" and the 2008 "I chose" HPV vaccine campaigns for Gardasil featured girls and young women addressing an audience of potential peers (Aronowitz 2010). A 2009 recap of the previous two campaigns showed pairs of mothers and daughters. Then, in October 2009, the Food and Drug Administration approved the quadrivalent HPV vaccine for males ages 9–26. A 2014 New York State vaccine awareness campaign—in the form of a brief video of a girl in a swing—addressed a generic genderless parent who was reminded that the vaccine was suitable for both girls and boys. The video ended with the claim that "HPV vaccine is cancer prevention" without reference to a specific type of cancer. The inclusion of boys and men in HPV vaccination awareness campaigns became explicit in Merck's 2016 "Who knew" advertising for—this time—an unnamed HPV vaccine. The video included actor portrayals of a girl and a boy, looking directly to the camera and reproachfully and rhetorically asking their "Mom" and "Dad" whether they knew about the life-saving vaccine. The campaign was linked to the website hpv.com, whose home page, as of November 2021, featured a mother with her son, a father with his daughter, another mother with her daughter, and three mothers together, with actors representative of White, Hispanic, and Black communities. In 2018, Merck introduced the HPV health literacy campaign, "Versed," whose website featured teen boys and girls of all races.

In Romania, the HPV vaccine remained exclusively feminine. The information campaign was launched after the first wave of vaccination failure, in January 2009 (see interlude, part 1), and featured the photo-image of a mother and her look-alike prepubescent daughter wearing matching white outfits and smiling at the camera (figure 6). On the bright red background, perhaps an allusion to

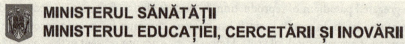

MINISTERUL SĂNĂTĂȚII
MINISTERUL EDUCAȚIEI, CERCETĂRII ȘI INOVĂRII

Tu decizi pentru sănătatea fiicei tale.
Informează-te!
O campanie a Centrului Național de Informare
pentru prevenirea cancerului de col uterin.

CENTRUL
NAȚIONAL
DE INFORMARE
PENTRU
PREVENIREA
CANCERULUI
DE COL UTERIN

TELVERDE:
08008-00008

Cancerul de col uterin este o boală ce poate afecta femeile de orice vârstă și reprezintă a doua cauză de cancer la femeile sub vârsta de 45 ani din întreaga lume. De aceea, ca mamă, ai dreptul de a fi corect informată înainte de a lua o decizie pentru copilul tău.

Intră pe www.informarehpv.ro

FIGURE 6. The feminization of HPV: Health Ministry poster for the HPV and cervical cancer awareness campaign. (Source: www.informarehpv.ro.)

the transition from girlhood to womanhood, the slogan in white, bold font suggested the pristine health that the vaccine was said to protect: "You decide for your daughter's health. Be informed!" (*Tu decizi pentru sănătatea fiicei tale. Informează-te!*) In October 2009, the National Federation of Parent Associations organized a debate about the HPV vaccine. When parents asked about the reasons for excluding boys from receiving the vaccine, the Health Ministry officials declared that vaccinating boys, while ideal, was not cost-effective.

Even though HPV is not a gender-specific infection, "the feminization of HPV" (Daley et al. 2017) is significant, as it aligns Romania with developing countries, where HPV vaccine campaigns have focused exclusively on girls and women. In an interview for GAVI (The Vaccine Alliance), founded by the Bill and Melinda Gates Foundation, Bill Gates himself only referenced girls in developing countries as potential beneficiaries of the vaccine. An advertising video produced by the Cancer Foundation of India and featured on the American Cancer Society online platform similarly focused only on the health and well-being of Indian girls, explained by a teenager and her mother.

While the HPV vaccine is supposedly meant to improve women's health and well-being, it also "reinforces the long-held belief that women are responsible for reproductive healthcare in heterosexual partnerships" (Daley et al. 2017, 145). In Romania, boys and men have been excluded as potential recipients of the HPV vaccination or as fathers and decision-making agents on behalf of their daughters. This is not accidental. Capitalizing on men's multifaceted reproductive invisibility that I have already discussed in this chapter, the feminization of the vaccine perpetuates old patriarchal prerogatives for men. Medical intervention aimed at controlling reproduction and reproductive health is only intended for women's bodies, which are thus reinscribed within the values and practices of patriarchy. By excluding boys from receiving the HPV vaccine, the Romanian authorities promote new forms of postcommunist state patriarchy that produce the reproductively invisible men of tomorrow.

THE ABORTED ROMANIA

In an ironic twist to the notion of men's reproductive invisibility during communism, after 1989, the ones who have voiced public concerns about reproduction were mostly men.[14] The most powerful visual creations that denounce Ceaușescu's pronatalism were produced by men—Florin Iepan directed the documentary *The Children of the Decree* in 2005, while Cristian Mungiu directed the movie *4 Months, 3 Weeks and 2 Days* in 2007. In 2011, the total estimated number of abortions performed between 1958 and 2008 was made public. The number—22,178,906—represented more than the actual total population of Romania at that moment.[15] These statistics, revealing the extraordinary amplitude of a mass phenomenon taking place for decades, prompted male journalists to speak of "the aborted Romania" (*Romania avortată*) and to make references to aborted fetuses as "a whole nation who could have lived, but will never come into being" (Fumurescu 2011). Rather than considering abortion from the angle of its tangible consequences on individual women, Fumurescu endorses the biopolitical fiction of an aborted nation. The notion of "aborted Romania" is yet another typification of a nation-state understood as a cohesive, monolithic organism (see also Magyari-Vincze 2006). *Post-factum* and through men's eyes, Romania contemplates its failure in the "aborted Romania." Iepan, Mungiu, and Fumurescu are all "children of the decree."

CONCLUSIONS

Using a plurality of sources—state propaganda scripts, official documents outlining family and reproductive policies, ethnographic data on gender interactions, women's recollections of reproductive events, and men's claims about their involvement in reproduction—I have, in this chapter, located men in relation to women's reproduction. Despite being hidden, Romanian men have not been absent from reproduction. Their traditional patriarchal prerogatives were simultaneously promoted and challenged by the communist state and its pronatalist demographic policies. Especially during the Ceaușescu era, men became reproductively invisible. In the aftermath of communism, patriarchal values and practices are still woven in the fabric of social life. Moreover, patriarchal prerogatives that grant men reproductive invisibility continue to guide the promotion and delivery of reproductive health care, including cervical cancer prevention. By generating reproductively invisible men, the communist and postcommunist patriarchal regimes of reproduction have had lasting effects on women's sexual and reproductive well-being. If, as I showed in chapter 1, the ghosts of past reproductive policies still harm women's current reproductive health because of their persistence, men's invisibility can also be deciphered through the grammar of hauntology. Except that, in this case, it is men's spectral elusiveness rather than ghostly endurance that enhances women's sense of reproductive vulnerability. Subjected to antagonistic relations with their in-laws and deprived of men's reproductive solidarity, some women were left to explore their sexuality and reproductive health within the meanings made available by everyday forms of religious practice. As we shall see in chapter 3, lived religion has provided some women from Delcel with both a conceptual and a practical framework for coping with perceived reproductive vulnerability.

INTERLUDE

Cervical Cancer Prevention: A Romanian Odyssey (Part 1)

On December 6, 2008, a large crowd gathered inside the Holy Trinity Orthodox Cathedral in Sibiu, a city of 400,000 in central Romania, to listen to metropolitan bishop Laurenţiu deliver the Saint Nicholas homily. Wearing a white robe and a richly adorned gold miter, Laurenţiu evoked the episode from the saint's life when he had prevented a destitute father from prostituting his own daughters. By helping the impoverished parent—Laurenţiu argued—Saint Nicholas had safeguarded not only the young women's spiritual integrity but their physical health as well. The bishop then compared the hagiographic story to the government-led human papillomavirus (HPV) vaccination campaign. The analogy was obvious: The father coercing his daughters into immoral behavior was the Romanian government pressuring parents to accept the HPV vaccine on behalf of their daughters. If Saint Nicholas's intervention saved the daughters from sinful behavior, the Romanian Orthodox Church similarly had to preserve Romanian girls' purity by urging parents to refuse the HPV vaccine for their daughters. Bishop Laurenţiu continued his homily and challenged the alleged benefits of the vaccine. He cast doubt on the "enigmatic link" between HPV and cervical cancer, enumerated other presumed cervical cancer risk factors besides the human papillomavirus, and speculated about insufficient clinical trials and unknown side effects. The burden of vaccination decision-making would be too much for parents, he added. Laurenţiu concluded his homily—which, at this point, had completely abandoned any reference to Saint Nicholas and had become a virulent criticism of the HPV vaccination campaign—by suggesting alternative state-sponsored programs aimed at fighting pornography and promoting family values.[1]

Bishop Laurenţiu was among the first public voices to forcefully react to the HPV vaccination campaign that the Health Ministry had launched just a few weeks earlier, on November 24, 2008. The government had spent about $37 million from public funds on 330,000 vaccine doses aimed at vaccinating 110,000 girls between ages 9 and 10. The vaccines—Gardasil and Cervarix—were produced, respectively, by Merck and GlaxoSmithKline and were brought into Romania from the Netherlands and the United Kingdom. The original plan was to administer the vaccine through school medical practices, once parental approval had been secured. The vaccination campaign had been hastily planned, with a last-minute ordinance issued by the Minister of Health and the President of the National Health Insurance House on October 20. The ordinance amended the 2008 immunization budget and immunization calendar to accommodate the HPV vaccination campaign.[2] In preparation for the campaign's kickoff, the online news platform HotNews.ro published an interview with epidemiologist Adrian Streinu-Cercel, the general manager of the National Institute for Communicable Diseases. When asked, "What should the mother of a ten-year-old girl know about the vaccine?" Streinu-Cercel explained the HPV link to cervical cancer and the vaccine's immunization mechanism and provided crude cervical cancer incidence and mortality statistics. He also claimed that he had already vaccinated his own wife and daughters (Bărăscu and Florea 2008).

Just days after the campaign started, Health Ministry officials met with parents who were concerned about the HPV vaccination controversies worldwide, notably in the United States. The parents asked for more information about clinical trials, side effects, accountability in case of side effects, and the rationale behind vaccinating fourth graders. They also wondered about their children's future access to public care if they got HPV after refusing vaccination. Several parents questioned the moral authority of Streinu-Cercel, suspected of an undeclared conflict of interests because of his past affiliation with GlaxoSmithKline (Preoteasa 2008). The same day, journalist Vlad Petreanu posted online a reaction under the caption "Anti-cancer vaccine: fanatics vs. medicine."[3] Petreanu uncritically endorsed the framing of the vaccine as "anti-cancer" and dismissed hesitating parents as religious fanatics for questioning the vaccine's benefits. His rhetoric was surprising, given that during the meeting with the Health Ministry officials, parents articulated vaccination objections using the language and values of biomedicine. According to Petreanu, other parents had already rejected the HPV vaccination because they entrusted their daughters' lives and well-being to "God's will" instead of modern medicine. The journalist also blamed the ministry's poor communication about the vaccine and predicted—remarkably early—the HPV vaccination campaign's failure. Neither Petreanu nor metropolitan bishop Laurențiu, who days later would deliver his anti-vaccination homily, had any medical training. Yet, early during the vaccination campaign, they both voiced publicly influential opinions that quickly polarized the debate around the HPV vaccination.

Two months after the campaign kickoff, only 2,615 girls (2.57 percent of the fourth graders cohort) had received the vaccine (Neagu 2009; Crăciun and

Băban 2012), which prompted the new Social-Democrat Minister of Health to suspend, in January 2009, the vaccination program launched by his Liberal predecessor. Blaming the campaign's initial results on the lack of communication about cervical cancer and HPV, the government created the National Information Center for Cervical Cancer Prevention (*Centrul Național de Informare pentru Prevenirea Cancerului de Col Uterin*, or CNIPCCU). CNIPCCU had a website and a toll-free phone line to facilitate access to information about cervical cancer and HPV. The pharmaceutical companies providing the vaccine sponsored an information campaign, launched on June 15, 2009, that featured pamphlets, posters, and video testimonials. These materials, designed for epidemiologists, family doctors, and school doctors, and for parents, professors, and children/students, were made available through medical practices, television, journals, and the Health Ministry and CNIPCCU websites.

In October 2009, the National Federation of Parent Associations organized a debate about the HPV vaccine, featuring special guest Streinu-Cercel, who explained again the link between HPV and cervical cancer. He endorsed the vaccine as "an investment in the future." The event also included the testimony of a young female journalist, Sanda Nicola, who was later featured in the HPV information campaign as well. Nicola shared her experiences as a cervical cancer survivor, promoted access to information, and criticized the Orthodox priests for their opposition to the HPV vaccine. "We are all at risk," she concluded. Other participants to the debate were an oncologist from Bucharest and a Health Ministry counselor. The oncologist pointed to the connection between cervical cancer incidence and poverty. The counselor provided an update on the information campaign and announced its next step, a professional survey of 1,000 parents on attitudes about vaccination. The counselor also acknowledged that the parental opt-out option was as an error. The plan was to replace it with a simple "no show."

A month later, the Health Ministry organized a press conference to communicate the results of surveying a sample of 1,044 parents of girls between the ages 12 and 14 about the HPV vaccination. The officials did not explain the survey methodology and the recruitment strategy. They claimed that 76 percent of parents had "a clear intention" regarding vaccination. However, this number appeared to have been miscalculated by adding the percentage of those who agreed to vaccination, not out of total but out of those who expressed a decision (52 percent), to the percentage of those who said they needed more information (24 percent). It was unclear how many parents expressed a decision. Also, asking for more information does not translate into a "clear intention." No additional data were released, despite the formal request by one member of the parliament. During the press conference, it was revealed that 8,000 doses had been administered to date, but it was unclear how many of these accounted for the second and third required shots. Based on the survey, the ministry decided to relaunch the HPV vaccination on November 23, 2009, exactly one year after the first failed campaign.

The start of the second HPV vaccination was eventually postponed to February 2010. This time, the campaign was aimed at a different age group: girls between ages 12 and 14. About a year later, in January 2011, media accounts about thousands of expired HPV vaccine doses started to emerge. And like the first, the second HPV vaccination campaign turned out to be a "total failure."[4] The Health Ministry, however, remained silent about the vaccination campaign outcome. Another two years later, during the European Week for Cervical Cancer Prevention in January 2013, Romanian Health Ministry representatives announced their plans for a third round of HPV vaccination starting March 2013, targeting girls between ages 10 and 14. A few weeks later, on February 4, Robb Butler, a specialist in health promotion, communication, and advocacy at the World Health Organization (WHO) visited Romania to share his expertise about how to start (!) an information campaign about the HPV vaccination. The third vaccination campaign was postponed until October 2013. In the meantime, the CNIPCCU website was deactivated. Between 2014 and 2020, the HPV vaccination program stalled, with no official updates from the ministry.

Occasionally, interest in vaccination fleetingly reemerged in the public eye. This was the case in January 2016, when several doctors signed a petition asking the government to resume the HPV vaccination campaign. In 2018, twenty-seven-year-old journalist Cecilia Laslo published a lengthy account documenting her attempts to get vaccinated against HPV (Laslo 2018). Her OB-GYN encouraged her to get the vaccine. Because she was past the age targeted for vaccination in Romania, Laslo was expected to buy herself all three doses of the HPV vaccine and to pay for it out-of-pocket at the pharmacy. At Laszlo's insistence, her family doctor wrote a prescription for the vaccine but refused to inoculate her because of the medical practice's policy to not administer vaccines brought by patients. After inquiring over the phone at several private clinics, Laslo finally found one clinic that agreed to administer the first dose of the HPV vaccine that the journalist would provide. Buying the vaccine proved an almost impossible task that Laslo accomplished only after checking in with tens of pharmacies in Bucharest. She eventually found the coveted vaccine and paid for the first dose the approximate equivalent of $160. On a hot summer day, Laslo took the HPV vaccine vial, carefully wrapped in ice by the pharmacist, and ran to the private clinic, where she was greeted by a nurse who, despite the information that the journalist had received earlier over the phone, was unwilling to administer the vaccine. After long negotiations, during which the ice started to melt, making the vial almost unusable, the still-grumpy nurse carelessly vaccinated Laslo in her hip. The needle—designed for vaccinating smaller prepubescent bodies—stopped in the fatty tissue, completely missing the muscle. One year later, Laslo emigrated to Norway, where she was included in a catch-up HPV vaccination campaign for adult women (Laslo 2019).

In contrast with the realities documented by Laslo, in the most recent development, on January 16, 2020, the Health Ministry published a press release about a seminar of medical experts discussing ways to increase trust in the HPV vaccine. In a major downsizing of the HPV vaccination campaign for 2020, the ministry distributed nationwide 20,000 doses for girls between ages 11 and 14 and, for 2021, 40,000 doses for girls between ages 11 and 18 whose parents had required vaccination—a far cry from the 330,000 doses of HPV vaccine that the government had bought more than a decade earlier. As of October 2021, only about 13,000 doses out of 40,000 had been used.

While the HPV vaccine became available as a form of primary prevention against cervical cancer less than two decades ago, secondary prevention in the form of Pap screenings has been routinely available worldwide since the 1960s (Hakama et al. 2008; Maver et al. 2013). The Papanicolaou smear test (abbreviated Pap) is a procedure in which cells from the cervix are collected and screened for abnormalities. The test can diagnose preinvasive and early invasive forms of cancer (Murthy and Landford Smith 2010, 269). The most current guidelines for "average risk women" between ages 21 and 65 recommend one Pap smear every three years. Women over age 30 are also advised to undergo HPV molecular cotesting every five years using the same swab as for the Pap test (CDC 2021).

Romania started its first national-scale cervical cancer screening program only in 2012 (Andreassen et al. 2017), but Pap tests had been administered to Romanian women for decades. Between 1967 and 1989, when the communist government enforced pronatalist policies, opportunistic cervical cancer screenings were sometimes part of mandatory gynecological controls. After 1989, there was a decline in cancer prevention programs due to a chronically underfinanced and mismanaged medical system. By 2006, the number of opportunistic Pap smears plummeted by a factor of seven compared to pre-1990 levels (Maver et al. 2013). Eventually, acquiescing to the European Union's pressures to align Romania's cancer prevention to global standards, the government created a cervical cancer prevention and control program (Apostol et al. 2010). In 2000, the Cancer Commission of the Health Ministry initiated local cervical cancer screening pilot programs. A year later, the programs were expanded at the regional level for Cluj County and, by 2004, covered several other counties of northwestern Romania (Apostol et al. 2010). In 2003, Romania joined the European Cancer Health Indicator Project (EUROCHIP), a European Union–financed survey of cancer incidence and mortality. Subsequent projects ran between 2003 and 2007 (EUROCHIP-2) and 2009 (EUROCHIP-3) (Apostol et al. 2010; Arbyn et al. 2010). In urban areas, family physicians would refer all women between ages 25 and 65 for Pap screenings. In rural areas, women were tested from a mobile unit. Cluj County joined in 2006 another European project of cancer data standardization, the European Network for Information on Cancer (EUNICE). A decline in incidence was noted after the implementation of pilot and regional screenings programs (Apostol et al. 2010). Finally, after years of planning and preparations, in 2012 the government started the first national screening program, with a reported coverage rate of 62.4 percent for the northwestern region (Maver et al. 2013). Additional Pap screening campaigns were launched in ten administrative regions throughout Romania. The program was considered a success by the Health Ministry officials, with a reported 40,000 women tested.

Yet, especially in peri-urban and rural areas, cervical cancer prevention campaigns did not significantly increase the number of women who received Pap tests. A competing narrative of rather intermittent access to reproductive care and cervical cancer prevention emerges from sociological surveys that challenge the reassuring official reports (see also Andreassen et al. 2017). A 2002 survey by the Romanian Center for Health Policies and Services revealed that, out of more than 700 women over eighteen years old, only 14 percent declared having had at least one Pap smear. Thirteen percent of them had never heard of the Pap test, while 73 percent had heard of it but claimed that they had never had one (MMT 2002). A 2005 study on cervical cancer screening reported that, out of more than 1,000 surveyed women, 31.5 percent and 20.8 percent had not had a gynecological control in the previous five and three years, respectively. Almost 10 percent of women were unable to recall the date of their last gynecological exam (Băban et al. 2005, 28). A report by the National Institute for Public Health showed that in 2006, only 8 percent of Romanian women had a Pap smear in the last year, by far the smallest percentage in Europe. Neighboring Bulgaria had an average of 15 percent, while the European Union average was 41 percent (Sănătate RO 2011). Another study from 2011 found that, among forty-two women with advanced cervical cancer, 61.11 percent declared never having been screened (Irimie et al. 2011).

In the most recent cervical cancer prevention development to date, the Health Ministry acquired in August 2018 eight mobile clinics intended to provide Pap tests to underserved populations starting with 2019. As of November 2021, no updates about the mobile clinic testing activity were available. In April 2021, the Health Ministry published the results of a recent reproductive health survey. Out of the 77 percent of the surveyed women who knew what the Pap screening was, 60 percent did not have one in the last three years (Cucu 2020).

3 · BEYOND RATIONALITIES

Bogdaproste! Bogdaproste! Bogdaproste!

Exclamations of gratitude pierce the indistinct humming of the crowd. It's early April, a cold and cloudy Friday afternoon, and the cemetery of Delcel is unusually animated. Dozens of women and children walk back and forth in apparent chaos on the narrow and muddy footpaths cut between the graves. Once in a while, they stop at particular graves at which women burn incense. Most adults carry plastic bags full of cheap candies that they distribute freely to everybody crossing their way. Upon receiving the sweets, children utter a high-pitched *Bogdaproste!* and continue to move along the path. I have come to the cemetery with Ileana, her grandchildren, and her neighbor, forty-eight-year-old Adriana, to participate to the Remembrance of the Dead, held each year on Good Friday. Ileana has brought an empty sardine tin can whose open lid is still partly attached to its rimmed edge. From her jacket pocket she extracts two handkerchief-wrapped bundles. She unwraps them carefully, displaying a few small pieces of frankincense and a couple of charcoals. Ileana places the charcoals inside the can and ignites them with a match. When the charcoals start to burn, she adds the incense. Holding the container by its semi-attached lid, she starts to move around her parents' twinned graves so that the musky smoke shrouds the funeral stones. The smoke is thick, black, and stifling; it bears little resemblance to the sweet-scented white incense fumes that Orthodox priests burn in the censer during church services. Meanwhile, Ileana's grandchildren are setting off a candy-collecting expedition around the cemetery. I leave Ileana by her parents' graves and escort Adriana to her father's burial place just a few yards away. On our way there, we give and receive sweets and exchange exclamations of *Bogdaproste!* Adriana tells me that saying a simple "thank you" (*mulțumesc*) would not be appropriate because we give and receive candies on behalf of the deceased, as alms for their dormant souls (*pomană de sufletul mortului*). *Bogdaproste* expresses acceptance of the gift in the name of the dead. Adriana burns charcoals and incense in a small single-handle urn and fumigates her father's grave (figure 7). Meanwhile, Ileana's grandchildren have returned with their pockets and hands full of bonbons, and we are ready to head back home.

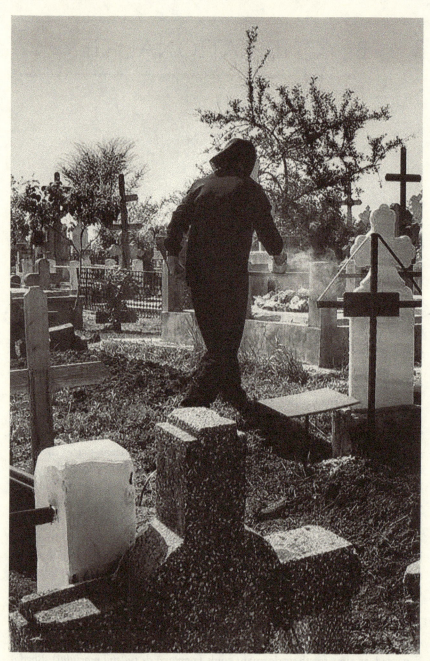

FIGURE 7. Woman burning incense on Good Friday in Delcel cemetery. (Photo by Pavel Bardă. Reprinted with permission.)

The Good Friday grave fumigation and sweets exchange is a ritual to remem-
the dead that the Orthodox Church neither officially endorses nor firmly condemns.
Voices within the church acknowledge that these memorials do not follow the canon
and express concerns about the improvised techniques of burning incense that alter
the quality—and, presumably, the purifying properties—of the smoke. Nevertheless, the Good Friday Remembrance of the Dead has been carried on every year,
along with other rituals that, although not strictly adhering to the Orthodox canon,
are imbued with religious meanings. Most of the women who shared with me their
reproductive life histories considered themselves active Orthodox worshippers.
They observed the official Orthodox celebrations and fasting days, venerated icons,
and attended liturgical services. But they also engaged in more informal rituals
that would better be described as "lived religion"—that is, "an ever changing, multifaceted, often messy—even contradictory—amalgam of beliefs and practices that
are not necessarily those religious institutions consider important" (McGuire 2008,
4; see also Hann and Goltz 2010). Compared with the sanctioned Orthodox rituals,
lived religious experiences appear as impure as the incense smoke from Ileana's
improvised censer. Nevertheless, the practical syncretism of lived religion informs
many aspects of the lives of Delcel women, in both ideology and action, even more
than the canonical Orthodox practice. That includes their views on sexuality and
reproduction, and their quest for reproductive health care.

In this chapter, I examine the local moralities that shape the sexual and reproductive lives of women from Delcel, as part of the series of systemic contingencies leading to Romania's cervical cancer crisis. Specifically, I look at how women
mobilize lived religion—as both discourse and grounding reality—as a decision-
making resource in contexts of perceived reproductive vulnerability. In chapters 1 and 2, I set the context of Romania's cervical cancer problem in relation
to the historical trauma produced by past repressive demographic policies,
respectively to forms of loneliness and reproductive vulnerability embedded in
patriarchal relations. In the following three chapters, I consider cervical cancer
in relation to the political economy of health care delivery, structural violence,
stratified reproduction, and uneven access to medical care resources. In this
chapter, however, I temporarily pause both historical and critical medical anthropology perspectives. I take up suggestions from nonsecular medical anthropology, a field of knowledge that "traces how all entities are both constructed and
real" and "would insist that when deities are part of medical practice, they are
integral to analysis" (Roberts 2016, 209). Here, I explore cervical cancer by integrating its nonsecular dimension, as revealed in women's experiences situated at
the intersection of lived reproduction and lived religion.

In chapter 2, I highlighted the extent to which many women's lives are shaped by
patriarchal relations that often entail female antagonism. As daughters-in-law,

Ileana, Maria, and others were excluded from networks of gender and kin solidarity when they were subjected to domestic violence and forced into using abortion as birth control. As I show in this chapter, rather than relying on their female (or male) relatives' advice and support, Oana, Maria, Ileana, Adriana, Tereza, and other women from Delcel mobilized lived religion to validate their reproductive decisions. Most of these women made use of noncanonical versions of Orthodox notions—such as God's will, godparenting, redemption, afterlife, and sin—to cope with their perceived reproductive vulnerability. As a reproductive decision-making resource, lived religion empowered them to navigate the complexities and paradoxes of conception and contraception, miscarriage and abortion, pregnancy and birth, and sexual and reproductive pathologies, including cervical cancer.[1] Juxtaposing such diverse sexual and reproductive events under a nonsecular umbrella only partly accounts for their particular contexts. Yet, women's experiences surrounding conception, abortion, and other reproduction events reveal broader ideas about the role that lived religion plays in shaping women's experiences of lived reproduction. To grasp the ways in which the nonsecular affects women's understanding of cervical cancer and its prevention, we need to consider a whole constellation of beliefs and practices that relate more generally to female sexuality and reproduction.

GOD'S WILL: CONCEPTION, ABORTION, CANCER

One July afternoon, I join Ileana on her way to Maria's place to drop off empty propane tanks. We take turns, pushing a heavy wheeled cart filled with tanks along the dusty, unpaved road. We find Maria busily weeding her tomato garden. She invites us both inside. We drink room-temperature store-bought lemonade. Aware of my interest in reproductive health care, Ileana deliberately brings into the conversation some gossip that has circulated in the neighborhood for a while. It is a tragicomical account of a Roşiorii de Vede gynecologist who has allegedly misdiagnosed a mother's premenopausal pregnancy for uterine cancer. (I analyze this urban legend in chapter 6). Maria laughs, Ileana gives me the look of an accomplice, and I seize the opportunity to discuss gynecological cancers and health care. When I ask Maria whether she has ever heard about the Papanicolaou test, the following conversation ensues:

MARIA: No, I haven't.

ILEANA: Me neither. I barely know what it's all about . . . well, I actually know something, but I never had one done!

MARIA: How is it called? Papa how?

CP: Papanicolaou. It is a test made on the cervix's cells that could detect cervical cancer.

MARIA: Do not do this to yourself! [It is] their cancer! I couldn't care less about cancer! Don't you see? It is God's will! Everybody plays [a role], poor, punished [people]. Let's not talk anymore about the world's punishment! [să nu mai vorbim de câtă pedeapsă e pe viața lumii]

When Maria confessed to her ignorance about the Pap test, Ileana also claimed that she knew little about the Pap smear and that she never had one. However, Ileana later admitted to me that her statement was not accurate. She understated her knowledge of cervical cancer prevention in a respectful attempt to make her senior neighbor Maria feel comfortable about her professed unfamiliarity with the test. Also, although Maria seemed oblivious to the Pap smear, this did does not necessarily mean that she never had one during her time as an unskilled factory laborer in the 1970s, under Ceaușescu's pronatalist regime, when gynecological controls—which sometimes included Pap smears (Kligman 1998, 154)—were forced on women. Regardless of Ileana's and Maria's actual or fabricated ignorance about the Pap smear, once I explained the purpose of the test, Maria became adamant in rejecting it. She drew on references from Christian imaginary about the Last Judgment and looked at cancer as a punishment for humans' flawed lives. Cancer was to her an expression of "God's will" (voia Domnului), a divine punitive intervention. As it became clearer from subsequent conversations, Maria applied a dual—secular and nonsecular—logic to her understanding of a woman's sexual and reproductive life. She saw all lived reproduction—from conception, birth, and abortion to pathologies such as breast or cervical cancer—as shaped, on the one hand, by a woman's ability to navigate patriarchal bargains with her husband or male partner and, on the other hand, by God's will.

Many of the women who shared their reproductive life histories with me also ascribed God's will an essential role in the onset of (reproductive) cancers, but also in conception and even in abortion as a means of birth control. They viewed conception as the result of summoning God's intervention through prayers, followed by sexual intercourse between partners.[2] The logic of these two steps to conception was that prayers would activate God's will, which would then reroute aimless sexuality into fruitful reproduction. The most senior women, Veturia (age 87) and Maria (age 74), went as far as to claim that praying to God for a baby was the only real prerequisite for conception. The notion of divine intervention for conception allows women to harmlessly link sexuality to motherhood—a crucial point of reconciliation, given that, in this region of southern Romania, motherhood is celebrated while a woman's sexuality is rather shrouded in silence and even shamed. To these women, summoning God's will to enable conception conveniently solves the patriarchal issue of impure female sexuality. Furthermore, divine intervention into conception dissociates, at least in part, conception from the body. On this basis, some women operated a discursive twist and invoked God's will in relation to abortion as well. Since conception occurs both inside and outside the body, abortion also happens only partly to a women's body and, by extension, to herself. Post-factum, some women tackled the somewhat paradoxical idea that abortion was also a manifestation of God's will of not letting some babies to be born. The lived religious understanding of divine intervention stages both conception and abortion as partially disembodied reproductive events.

Besides conception and abortion, women also saw cancer as a partly disembodied experience. Almost half of the women who talked to me[3] acknowledged environmental pollution or the consumption of additive-laden foods as potential causes of cancer, but they still considered cancer an expression of God's will, overpowering any human attempt to control the life course. Although Maria was the only one to urge *me* not to have a Pap test, throughout my time in Delcel, I carried out fourteen similar conversations about cervical screening with women who were either indifferent about the test or even expressed blunt refusal to undergo it. Significantly, all of these women were over age 45. Many were aware that the screening was available free of charge with a referral from the family doctor.

Women's rejection of free preventive care that could potentially diagnose a life-threatening condition may seem counterintuitive. As I was struggling to not romanticize or exoticize women's decision-making strategies, at first I hypothesized that some of them did not understand the link between being tested and possibly being diagnosed. The prosaic predictability of insufficient health literacy was a plausible explanation. Yet, on many occasions, I had witnessed Roşiorii de Vede residents engaging in savvy tactics of navigating medical care. It was unlikely that their presumed lack of health literacy had prevented women from undergoing cervical screening. As experienced ethnographers established, time and again, people's claims rarely if ever completely overlap with their actual life experiences. After all, the dialogue about the Pap test with an oblivious Maria— who may unknowingly have had the test in the past—and a politely deceitful Ileana—who claimed ignorance about the test—demonstrate the elusive character of such conversations. To clarify whether women understood the link between cervical screening and cervical cancer detection, I reviewed my field notes and interview transcripts and conducted brief follow-up interviews. Most women from Delcel understood that early detection testing could diagnose cancer. In only three cases, Maria's included, I had to explain what a Pap smear was. Women did recognize the connection between cervical screening and cervical cancer detection, but they chose to dismiss its relevance.

What women from Delcel declined to acknowledge by revealing God's will as the ultimate trigger of cancer was not the causal connection between the Pap test and cervical cancer detection. To them, the conversation was not even about cancer prevention; it was instead about their perceived sense of embodied reproductive vulnerability. My questions about the Pap smear forced some women to reconsider personhood through the lens of preventive medicine. Their rejection of the cervical screening translated a refusal to envision themselves as "presymptomatic persons" (Konrad 2005) whose bodies are scrutinized for invisible pathologies. This refusal of the presymptomatic as the very principle of preventive medicine can also be deciphered from a hauntology perspective. In the end, what women resisted was the specter of the disease lurking around.

The notion of divine predestination encapsulated in God's will intersects with preventive medicine's narratives of risk. Practices as diverse as Nuer divination, Siberian shamans' trance, and predictive genetics readings all turn bodies into oracles (Konrad 2005; Lock and Kaufert 1998; Evans-Pritchard [1937] 1976). Invoking God's will to justify the refusal to engage in cervical cancer prevention is, like cervical testing itself, a form of anticipating pathological bodies. However, that divine predestination and biomedical risk are not isomorphic notions is proved when the women of Delcel privilege the nonsecular definitions of personhood and ground their rejection of cervical cancer prevention in a lived religion's understanding of the ways God's will shapes human life. Women's reservations should be understood against the background of a nonsecular decision-making process.

In addition to summoning God's will in relation to their own bodies and health, women also entrusted their daughters' and granddaughters' well-being to divine intervention, as revealed during our conversations about the human papillomavirus (HPV) vaccination.

Amalia works as a cashier at a newly opened supermarket. She grew up in a nearby village and, when she was fourteen years old, moved to the boarding school of the best high school in Roșiorii de Vede. A bright student, Amalia passed her high school graduation exam (baccalaureate) with flying colors and was admitted at the university in Bucharest. However, on pressure from her family, she married a railroad engineer the same summer and gave up university. She moved in with her in-laws in Delcel. At thirty-four, Amalia is the mother of twelve-year-old Tina. Her daughter was included in the target population to receive the HPV vaccine, but Amalia opted out. Eager to talk about the vaccination campaign, Amalia has invited me over at her house. It is a mild and sunny October afternoon. I stop in front of a massive metal gate that hides the house and the yard. I ring the bell and Tina, a blue-eyed girl, all smiles, opens the gate and guides me through a concrete alley. The courtyard is covered with sweet-scented grapevines. We pass by a chicken coop that smells pungent from bird droppings. Slightly nauseous from the mixture of smells, I am let in. Tina vanishes. Amalia and I are sitting in the living room, drinking Nescafé instant coffee. We can overhear the five o'clock news that her mother-in-law watches on a small TV in the nearby kitchen.

I won't accept this vaccine for my girl. As long as she is a virgin, I will not take any action. I don't want to trigger side effects and ruin her body and health. I don't want to cry later over my wrong choice. It's better to let things follow their normal way and not to tamper with God's will.

Amalia associates the "normal way" with "God's will." She implies that human life is ultimately governed by divine predestination and that medical intervention is somehow artificially shaping alternative bodies and lives. Yet, Amalia's invocation of "God's will" seems to be a hopeful one, where divine predestination is assumed to mostly be divine protection. "God's will," she presumes, is that her daughter would simply be protected without any preventive care. (In chapter 6, I consider again Amalia's statement from a different perspective.)

More than a dozen women from Delcel explicitly mentioned God's will to explain their refusal to allow their daughters and granddaughters to receive, in the near or distant future, the HPV vaccine. They implied, once again, that cervical cancer etiology is, at least in part, beyond human control. With the exception of Maria, who explicitly claimed that cancer was a punishment for the world's sins, other women did not identify the cause of (cervical) cancer as a moral breach. However, the women did not regard the human papillomavirus as the solely trigger of the condition. They rather emphasized the crucial role of the divine logic—that escapes rationality—in the onset of the (cervical) cancer. Furthermore, God's will was not only the ultimate cause of cervical cancer, but also its only cure. According to fifty-nine-year-old Tinca, grandmother to nine-year-old Felicia, "When you got the [HPV] virus, you have nothing left but God."

THE MORALITIES OF LIVED REPRODUCTION

During the pronatalist era and beyond, women's reproductive experiences have been at odds with both secular and religious moralities. State authorities and the Romanian Orthodox Church (BOR) (figure 8) regulate reproduction from, respectively, the biopolitics and the bioethics perspectives. But in the end, both state and church ignore the lived realities of reproduction. The fact that, over the last seven decades, women have continued to use abortion as a method of birth control despite both secular and nonsecular restrictions points to the persistence of tactics of staging abortion as a reasonable everyday practice. I suggest that lived religion has assisted women in meaningfully processing not only abortions but also an entire constellation of sexual and reproductive events, including cervical cancer and its prevention.

In addition to summoning God's will in relation to their sexual and reproductive health, some women from Delcel articulated their perceived sense of reproductive vulnerability by exploring—in both discourse and practice—noncanonical versions of other Orthodox ideas. For instance, they justified abortion as birth

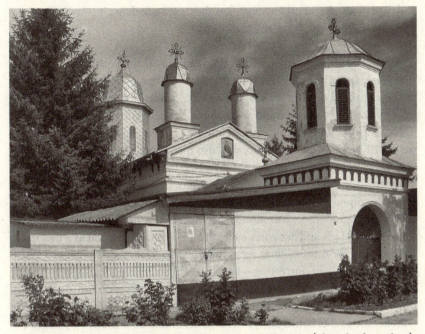

FIGURE 8. Saint Elias church of Delcel district in Roşiorii de Vede. (Photo by the author.)

control by mobilizing "unorthodox" versions of the Orthodox notions of god-parenting, redemption, afterlife, and sin. Women's abortion stories were imbued with alternative religious meanings that, once elaborated, were expanded on everything relating to reproduction and reproductive health. To better understand how women integrated the nonsecular in their perceptions about cervical cancer and its prevention, it is thus useful to consider the ways they instrumentalized religious tropes in explaining abortion as birth control. Their accounts provide a thicker ethnographic context to an analysis of more general views about reproductive health, including cervical cancer.

Her reproductive years long gone, Maria recalls her numerous abortions on a lamenting tone: "I did not have one abortion, I had thirty! Oh, Miss Cristina, thirty I had! Oh, God, may God forgive us, and may [God] spare us the punishment to eat them all [fetuses], once we reach the afterlife." Maria pauses, visibly distraught. She crosses herself several times before resuming, in a higher pitch voice:

'Cause you know what? [My husband] was drunk all the time and I was tired and vulnerable, taking care of animals, of cows, of devils. He had mistresses and fiddlers playing to him, all day long, drunk. And I had two, three [babies] every year, but I went to the doctor and expelled them. I didn't go to old sage women, I had doctor S. and this other one . . . the old and short one. Then they were not allowed [to perform abortions] anymore, but they were still doing it secretly. So, I was getting [abortions]. What else to do?[4]

Maria had these abortions from the late 1950s through the early 1970s. As noted in chapter 1, during this time period, the communist state's reproductive policies changed drastically, with the sudden criminalization of abortion stipulated by Decree 770 in 1966 and an unofficial ban on modern contraception. The decree was promulgated by atheist authorities to increase natality and expand the future working-class generation. I also mentioned that Decree 770 did not stop women—Maria included—from seeking to terminate their pregnancies on a fast-growing market of clandestine abortions. In a rural and peri-urban Romania with cultural roots in traditional patriarchy and virtually no access to modern contraception, abortion had already been used as a method of birth control. Women like Maria and her peers have consistently used abortion as a method of birth control for most of their reproductive years (Johnson, Horga, and Fajans 2004). Although disconcerting—because of the very high number of claimed abortions—Maria's personal history of repeated abortions is similar to millions of other stories of Romanian women. Yet, Maria's confession is far from ordinary. She links her use of abortion as birth control to her husband's discretionary exercise of sexual prerogatives. As a response to the disempowering circumstances of repeated marital rape, abortion appears justified to Maria. However, because of the Orthodox stance that abortion is a sin, she expresses concern about future punishment. In Maria's view, abortion is redeemable in the afterlife through a dreadful cannibalistic act (see also Sasson and Law 2009). The meanings of fetal cannibalism are double-fold. First, a woman is forced to ingest the aborted fetuses to literally undo their premature expulsion. Second, the sinner has to engage in one of the most atrocious and dehumanizing actions—that of eating human flesh.

Like many of her peers from southern rural Romania, Maria is an active Orthodox worshipper, but the way she sees abortion—as both practice and ideology—has little to do with the official views on the topic, as expressed by the Romanian Orthodox Church. To address the moral transgressions of her lived reproduction experiences, she mobilizes lived religion and imagines a non-canonical yet religious version of the afterlife that allows her to redefine, within a nonsecular semantics, abortion as a redeemable practice. Abortion-as-a-yet-to-redeem-sin provides narrative coherence to Maria's reproductive life history, as it links past, present, and future, and it allows her to even imagine the afterlife. As Maria's story suggests, lived religion may be a reproductive decision-making resource allowing some women to meaningfully articulate their lived reproduction experiences. In spite of past reproductive traumas, lived religion empowers women to envision the future.

Women who shared their stories with me did not express any particular concern about BOR's official condemnation of abortion. However, all of them perceived terminating a pregnancy as a sin—but a possibly redeemable one. Besides Maria, just a few others were concerned with afterlife punishments for abortion, but many more were preoccupied with practical ways of redemption in *this* life. They saw godparenting (*nășitul*) as the best way to redeem an abortion. Rather than focusing on the dogmatic condemnation of abortion, women chose to engage in lived religion practices rooted in enduring kin relations, either real or metaphorical. Women believe that when one assumes the godmother role and provides lifelong spiritual guidance and material support to another couple's child, she compensates for having had an abortion. Expanding kinship networks through godparenting rectifies the potential disruption in the descent line produced by the abortion. Reproduction is again understood as disembodied, as it shifts from individual bodies to the social body and from biological child-rearing to spiritual parenting.

During our conversations, I noted the lexical choices that women made when recounting their reproductive experiences. In southern Romania, the postpartum period is marked by naming taboos. During the first forty days of a newborn's life, until the baby receives the Orthodox christening, family members routinely avoid calling the baby by name, using instead metaphors—such as "sweet little bread" (*cozonăcel*) or "little loaf of bread" (*franzeluță*). Naming interdictions are meant to protect the fragility of a new life in an acknowledgment of the newborn's liminality. Some women used similar linguistic mechanisms to refer to their aborted fetuses. Their word choices attenuated rather than assigned personhood to the unborn. Veturia, an eighty-seven-year-old former factory inspector and mother of a unique son, bluntly explains: "I married very young and I was completely ignorant [about contraceptive methods]. I had no one to talk to. I did abort a whole soccer team." Veturia's intention in using the soccer team metaphor was to emphasize the high number of pregnancies that she had terminated, since a soccer team has eleven players, but she also imagined the fetuses, collectively, as a team. The aborted soccer team allegory reflects Veturia's avoidance to ascribe personhood to never born babies. Yet, even without individual characteristics, the aborted fetuses are gendered in her description. There is an underlying patriarchal connotation in her wording because in Romania, soccer is an exclusively masculine sport that stands for virility. Veturia's assumption that she had aborted male fetuses speaks about a patriarchal preference for sons over daughters. Similarly, other women from Delcel either referred to their aborted fetuses with collective nouns ("bunch," "pile," "team," or even "half of a team") or completely avoided any reference to the unborn and talked about abortion as a no-outcome event. These discursive strategies articulated, again, abortion as a partially disembodied reproductive experience.

While still upholding to the notion of abortion as a sin, some women chose to politicize the issue of pregnancy termination. If Maria professed the unavoidability of abortion as birth control, Oana articulates the need to access modern contraception as a moral right that should be granted by the secular state and endorsed through nonsecular education. To my question about the next steps a woman should follow once she realizes she is pregnant, Oana retorts: "If she intended to get pregnant, she must be happy. If she got pregnant accidentally, she should regret [it]. She could have taken contraceptive pills instead. Especially now that pills are allowed. In any case, she shouldn't consider having an abortion. No way."

Oana briefly pauses, before continuing in a crescendo: "I could have had four [children] instead of two. This is murder—it really is murder. There is life from conception and OB-GYNs are murderers! The state and health ministry should provide pills to all women, to all young girls, starting at fifteen. They should develop a campaign . . . for contraception because abortion is murder."

I tell Oana that many of her neighbors and acquaintances in Roşiorii de Vede and beyond would see making pills available on a large scale to young girls as problematic. But Oana has a solution: "This is where mothers play a role. This is why these girls have mothers, right? But, many times, mothers chose to stay away from this." I remind her that, from my conversations with older women from Delcel, I noticed that many of the mothers were raised during the communist times, with virtually no access to contraceptive education. Yet Oana believes in the value of mother–daughter dialogues: "Some talked to their daughters, told them abortion is not the way—it's a sin and [it's] dangerous. There are [mothers] like me, but there are many who just don't care."

Oana frames her claims of life from conception by using a selective reading of the Orthodox interdiction of abortion, abortive remedies, and modern contraception. In addition to balancing the pro-life and pro-choice discourses, Oana foresees a win–win partnership between state authorities and parents to solve the issue of abortion as birth control. As with other topics, her opinions are exceptional compared to those of her counterparts. While studies on mother–daughter communication about sexuality and reproduction are still missing in Romania, Oana's observation rings true. Whether from a religious or a secular perspective, especially in rural areas, mothers are reluctant to address such topics with their daughters.

UNDERSTANDING PREVENTION

In resource-poor countries, the focus is on curative medicine. Financial constraints and material shortages cast prevention as marginal. Here, a diagnosis of cancer can be received as a death sentence (McMullin et al. 2005). In Romania— a still-developing country by measure of its Human Development Index, with a mix of urban growth and rural poverty—ideas about cancer often revolve around its unavoidability (Crăciun and Băban 2012; Grigore et al. 2017). Romanians (and other southeast Europeans) are frequently portrayed as fatalistic about their health and well-being. Named "Balkanism," for the geographical area where these populations are spread (Todorova 1997), this worldview is characterized as a passive and noncombat psychology of "waiting for something to come from above" (Todorova et al. 2006, 781). Whether because of Balkanism or not, many Romanians tend to see cancer as a condition beyond human control. However, understanding cancer as an expression of an overpowering supernatural or unnatural force does not inevitably deter patients from seeking treatment. On the contrary, for some patients, faith provides an additional coping mechanism when facing a cancer diagnosis and undergoing treatment.

Behavioral psychology studies have considered Balkanism and religious and spiritual beliefs in relation to cancer diagnosis and treatment but not prevention (Bizo, Opre, and Rusu 2014). To date, there is only one large survey that documented, through a questionnaire administered at the doctor's office, awareness and knowledge about the Pap smear among 431 Romanian women from urban and rural areas (Grigore et al. 2017). More than 40 percent of them declared never having had a Pap test. Like many of the women from Roşiorii, the women in the study listed as screening barriers lack of time and money, feelings of embarrassment about the gynecological examination, perceived lack of need to be screened, and fatalistic attitudes related to cancer (Grigore et al. 2017).

Additionally, one qualitative methods investigation of cervical cancer screening in Romania and Bulgaria focused not on women's own understandings but on health care providers' perceptions about women's role in cervical cancer prevention (Todorova et al. 2006). According to the men and women OB-GYNs interviewed in the study, Romanian and Bulgarian women are "modernity deficient," "irresponsible," uninterested in taking care of their own health, and even "sexually promiscuous." Health care providers situate their prejudice against these women in a mainstream biomedical rationality that perpetuates stereotypical representations of undisciplined subjects. Women are misconstrued by doctors as lacking cancer prevention literacy. However, the women of Roşiorii de Vede are not oblivious to biomedicine's preventive solutions. Furthermore, if "modernity deficient" means privileging nonsecular rationalities in health care seeking tactics, these women are, in fact, "modern." I expected women to summon lived religion in their narratives about reproductive medicine and cervical cancer prevention. To my surprise—given that they repeatedly invoked the nonsecular in their descriptions of reproductive bodies, events, and pathologies—they did not even allude to religion in their comments about preventive reproductive care. There was almost no continuity between women's views about reproduction and reproductive bodies and their understandings of preventive reproductive care.

The inconsistency in invoking the nonsecular with respect to reproductive bodies but not in relation to preventive reproductive care may be explained by the ways Romanians remember the past, understand the present time, and imagine the future. In biomedicine, preventive care creates a temporal inversion. It suspends the *here and now* of the living body, replacing it with the specter of a future pathological body. Prevention is about imagining and taming the future. Yet, to the women from Delcel who are forty-five and older, prevention is intimately linked—historically and personally—to the past. As I show in greater depth in chapter 4, they associate preventive screening like the Pap test to the past historical regimes of mandatory gynecological controls and to their reproductive years now gone. Far from empowering these women to imagine a better and healthier future for themselves—and through the HPV vaccination, for their (grand)daughters as well—prevention reminds them about the traumas and failures of the past. In contrast, when it comes to imagining a hopeful future, most of them would rather rely on God's will than a state program. Whether on practical, spiritual, or other, more ambiguous grounds, enrolling or not into preventive sexual and reproductive care is the consequence of a decision-making process. I turn now to explore how women integrate secular and nonsecular ideas about female bodies, sexual and reproductive pathologies, and prevention into decision-making instruments when considering access to cervical cancer prevention.

"IRRATIONAL" DECISION-MAKING

Worldwide, the HPV vaccine has been advertised by portraying young girls as being "at risk" for cervical cancer (Wailoo et al. 2010). However, some parents and guardians challenged the biomedical framing of the vaccine as the best treatment against cervical cancer (Towghi 2010). The early debates about the HPV vaccine revolved around parental anxieties caused by the incomplete understanding of the relationship between the HPV and cervical cancer, allegations of insufficient laboratory testing before public implementation, apprehensions about short and long-term side effects, and uncertainties about the duration and efficacy of the immune protection conferred by vaccination (Wailoo et al. 2010; Coleman, Levison, and Sangi-Haghpeykar 2011; Haas et al. 2009; Connell and Hunt 2010). This list of issues tends to objectify responses rather than demonstrate their shifting qualities, but it is nevertheless useful in documenting the range of parental responses. In a 2012 study, Romanian mothers voiced similar concerns regarding the HPV vaccine as their counterparts worldwide (Crăciun and Băban 2012). In their narratives of vaccination refusal, women did not mention nonsecular objections to vaccination. Unlike the 2012 study, which was carried out in a large urban area among educated women, my research in Delcel reflects the knowledge, attitudes, and practices of rural and peri-urban women. The findings that I discuss in this chapter indicate how a large and understudied population frames cervical cancer prevention refusal.[5] Moreover, when corroborated with Crăciun and Băban's report, my research in Roșiorii de Vede suggests that women who live in urban areas are more likely to refuse HPV vaccination on medical and secular grounds than women from rural localities, with the latter more likely to invoke nonmedical and nonsecular reasons for HPV vaccination refusal.

Globally, HPV vaccine marketing targeted parents, and especially mothers, as decision-makers on behalf of their daughters (and later, in some countries, sons) and their future sexual and reproductive health. However, parental knowledge about and support for the HPV vaccination has been uneven. Some parents backed up their decisions about HPV vaccination with secular arguments while others invoked the nonsecular as well. In the United States, among the 609 mothers surveyed in North Carolina, 81 percent initiated vaccination discussions in order to help their daughters assess the future of their reproductive health (McRee et al. 2011). However, parents from Colorado rejected the HPV vaccine because they felt it removed a potential tool for teaching sexual responsibility to their teenage children. These parents "expect[ed] to remain central in their children access to health care" (Reich 2010, 178). In Brazil, 92 and 86 percent of 826 surveyed parents, respectively, supported the HPV vaccine for their daughters and sons (Mendes Lobão et al. 2018). In Peru, parental ambivalence about the HPV vaccine being administered to fifth graders slowed their decision-making process. Torn between perceived benefits and risks of vaccination, Peruvian parents sought additional information to consolidate their knowledge before consenting or opting out from the free immunization program (Bartolini et al. 2012). In Morocco, out of 670 mothers and 182 fathers, an overwhelming majority were not aware of the HPV vaccine, many did not know about the Pap test, and none had vaccinated their daughter(s). Moroccan parents largely agreed with the assertion that "whatever happens to my health is God's will" (Mouallif et al. 2014).

In Romania, after the first failed vaccination wave of 2008–2009, new marketing information about cervical cancer and HPV was broadcast to support the 2010–2011 HPV vaccination campaign. It failed to boost vaccination rates, however, in part because marketing misread mothers' self-perceived role as decision-makers in protecting the future reproductive well-being of their daughters. The mothers and grandmothers who talked to me about the HPV vaccination were reluctant to decide on behalf of their (grand)daughters.

It's a scorching late August afternoon. I have joined Monica (age 29), her daughter Felicia, and her mother Tinca in their wooden cabin—a pleasant refuge from the outside heat, since it is built on top of their backyard cellar. We are chatting while husking corn in the cool and dark cabin, surrounded by the floating dust of intermittently piercing sunny rays. Monica explains her refusal to allow her nine-year-old daughter to be vaccinated: "*Me* deciding for her? This is not right. This is playing God. . . . I don't play God!" Tinca, Felicia's grandmother, muses: "I am afraid to think for Felicia. How could *I* decide for her?" Tinca stresses the "I" in her rhetorical question.

Monica sees the HPV vaccine as an instrument that would allow her to wrongfully claim power over her daughter's life. The vaccine operates a moral disruption in a predestined order governed by divine will. Tinca also questions her agency regarding her granddaughter's health. By renegotiating "the moral values attached to human life" (Weiner 2009, 320), these women actively conveyed renewed definitions of personhood for themselves and for their (grand)daughter. Their perception of a divine logic scripting women's and girls' reproductive well-being provided them the moral ground to exert their veto.

Rather than perceiving the vaccine as an empowering tool, parents from Roşiorii contemplated the limits and the futility of prevention in shaping their daughters' yet-to-come reproductive lives. By addressing a presumed sense of parental agency, the HPV advertising campaign misconstrued the mothers and grandmothers and their right to determine their (grand)daughters' future health. Monica and Tinca delegated authority—at least in part—to forms of nonsecular agency like God's will. Although they asserted their skepticism about decision-making, the women who refused Pap testing or HPV vaccination had nevertheless made a firm decision not to let themselves or their (grand)daughters be part of these health promotion programs. The mothers and grandmothers from Delcel challenged biomedical assumptions about "normal" bodies and "standards" of reproductive health care embedded in cervical cancer prevention.

Women's lived experiences within the context of religion intersected with patriarchal understandings about gendered bodies to produce forms of "local biologies" (Lock and Nguyen 2010, 90; see also Lock 1993). Seen through the lens of local biologies, Delcel residents' responses to cervical cancer prevention recontextualized notions such as "mother love" (Scheper-Hughes 1992; Einarsdóttir 2000; Gottlieb 2004) and "irrational reproduction" (Krause and DeZordo 2012). In a well-known ethnographic example of people invoking God's will in relation to children's lives, Nancy Scheper-Hughes (1992) tells us how Brazilian shantytown mothers' "failure to mourn" their infants' deaths challenges universalistic assumptions about mother love. Catholic ideas of an afterlife where dead infants become guardian angels watching over the living help Brazilian mothers cope with child loss. Infant illness and death only prove the power of God's will (Scheper-Hughes 1992). In dialogue with Scheper-Hughes's findings, Jónína Einarsdóttir draws on fieldwork in Guinea-Bissau to defend a less intransigent position on provisional mother love. Einarsdóttir (2000, 6) finds that "cultural values and ethical considerations related to religion and kinship ideologies, as well as gender relations and subsistence are all important factors in shaping reproductive practices, and in turn maternal affection and dedication." My fieldwork findings concur, redefining mother love in contextual rather than absolute terms. For women of Delcel, lived religion validates, in discourse and practice, local definitions of mother love that do not necessarily include HPV vaccination acceptance.

Even if not explicitly articulated as moral or religious exemptions, women's assertions that their health and that of their daughters and granddaughters is ultimately conditioned by God's will amount, from a public health perspective, to "non-informed refusal" of medical intervention (Berlinger and Jost 2010, 206). That people would decline free preventive care that could either prevent or diagnose at early, curable stages a life-threatening condition is unintelligible from the perspective of biomedical rationality. Yet, with the increased medicalization of reproduction, instances of resistance to medical intervention—even if often fluid and partial—have multiplied (Davis-Floyd 2003; Fordyce and Maraesa 2012; Franklin and Ragoné 1998; Lock and Kaufert 1998; Ginsburg and Rapp 1995). I was reminded that "people constantly exceed the projections of experts" and that "the medicoscientific, political, humanitarian frameworks in which they are temporarily cast cannot contain them" (Biehl and Petryna 2013, 5). Anthropology has long been critical of mainstream "biomedical rationality," with researchers adding to our knowledge that people operate with multiple and competing rationalities of care, which are embedded in social, cultural, and religious institutions (Chapman 2010; Gottlieb 2004; Webster 2013). Popular explanations for disease, suffering, and death are multilayered (Lock and Nguyen 2010). Romanian women are not the only ones to invoke God's will instead of—and often in parallel with—seeking medical care (Flórez et al. 2009; Johnson 2006). Their refusal of cervical cancer prevention demonstrates that, in addition to a specific sense of reproductive vulnerability, there are local ethics of responsibility that are rooted in a morality of care that has precedence over the official rationalities of preventive medicine. I argue that, far from "irrational," this alternative morality of care operates through what I call "beyond rationalities"—practical reasoning that integrates both the secular and the nonsecular (see also Roberts 2012).

As I show in chapters 4 and 5, the postcommunist reforms of medical care have created emergent landscapes of health inequalities. Are Delcel residents' references to God's will discursive rationalizations of their anxieties about the changing definitions of adequate care? By relinquishing control over their own health to a force from beyond, do people express their feeling of disempowerment regarding access to health care resources?[6] I suggest that, on the contrary, invoking the nonsecular to decline cervical cancer prevention opens up a discursive space where resistance is explicitly articulated and reproductive control over one's body is reappropriated. References to God's will empower women to challenge what they perceive as state-driven reproductive control by making a counterintuitive yet bold choice. Lived religion allows women to display an ethos of asserting agency that is akin to a neoliberal tenet. Yet, the mere mention of God's will did not necessarily imply that women refused the HPV vaccination in the name of "laws, policies, and practices that explicitly concern adherence to religious doctrine" (Berlinger and Jost 2010, 197), as has happened, for instance, among faith-healing devotees in the United States. Questions arise about the interplay between religious faith, perceived vulnerability, lack of knowledge about the benefits of vaccination, and the practicalities of everyday life. A revealing case is the unexpected success of a family planning campaign among Catholic Mexican women who "proved far less religiously bound and more concerned with providing their fewer children with better educational opportunities and material privilege than some analysts has suspected possible" (Gutmann 2011, 63).

Did the mothers and grandmothers from Roșiorii de Vede delegate responsibility for preventive reproductive care for their daughters and granddaughters based on their Orthodox faith? Or, conversely, did they use nonsecular references to justify their refusal to act as decision-makers? In the absence of an official pronouncement regarding the HPV vaccination issued by the Romanian Orthodox Church,[7] women made use of God's will as a discursive strategy aimed at articulating their moral alienation from the state-driven medical intervention. Considering Romania's recent history of brutal intervention into women's reproduction, lived religion provided Delcel residents with a means for staging and voicing resistance to state medicine. However, living circumstances should not be reduced to discourse or social construction, "because the very possibility of discursive arguments comes from the reality of autonomous existence" (Roberts 2016, 216–217). God's will is more than a mere rhetorical device, since it correlates in many of these women's embodied reproductive experiences, as revealed through their lived religion narratives and practices about conception, contraception, abortion, and cervical cancer.

CONCLUSIONS

Many of the women who shared their reproductive life histories with me mobilized lived religion to make sense of their sexuality and reproduction. They linked conception, abortion as a method of birth control, and cervical cancer to forms of divine intervention that partially disembody human reproduction and its pathologies. While considered a serious sin, abortion can still be redeemed through social performances that transfer actual descent to spiritual kin relations through godparenting. Redemption for abortion can also be granted in a noncanonical afterlife. Language expresses the partial disembodiment of abortion, with women employing linguistic taboos to decline personhood to the unborn. Looking beyond biopolitical and bioethical conceptualizations of abortion as articulated by both state and church, and considering the nonsecular, allows us to better understand the ways that women have routinely framed abortion as contraception in the last seven decades. The nonsecular perspective on abortion may also explain, at least in part, the persistence of this practice of fertility control among Romanians. Unlike the state's and church's views on abortion, which settle the issue in unambiguous terms, everyday religious meanings and narratives have a correlate in women's actual reproductive experiences. As a decision-making resource, lived religion appears to empower some women to navigate the complexities of conception and contraception.

While cervical cancer is regarded by some as an expression of God's will, women do not always mobilize the nonsecular to explain cervical cancer prevention. In some instances, Delcel residents perceive biomedicine's normative approach as disrupting "the normal way" set out by God's will (recall Amalia's refusal of the HPV vaccine), while in other cases women simply privilege secular rationalities different from the official biomedical ones. People's responses to these prevention programs are diverse, mixing the secular and nonsecular.

On the one hand, in response to official biomedical narratives and practices such as the HPV vaccination, parents activate religious counternarratives that provide moral legitimacy to their refusal of medical care and empower them to take control over their daughters' bodies. Far from stripping ordinary citizens of their choices regarding access to reproductive health care, the nonsecular appears to constitute the very medium through which they display individual agency. On the other hand, women of Delcel did not summon lived religion when they rationalized their refusal to engage in preventive gynecological controls, such as having a Pap smear. As I show in more detail in chapter 4, in a temporal reversal, they associated preventive controls not with the promise of future health and well-being but with the historical and personal reproductive traumas of the past. Women mobilized the nonsecular to imagine a better future for their daughters and granddaughters, but they read the past in a rather secular key. The nonsecular medical anthropology approach has been useful in emphasizing localized resistance to cervical cancer prevention. However, women's secular responses compel us to turn toward the structural forces that concern critical medical anthropology. The suffering produced by past pronatalist policies, along with patriarchal understandings of female bodies, fashion women's secular ideas about the futility of engaging in cervical cancer prevention. In the end, it is control over one's body that outweighs health. The following chapters will highlight the ways in which the restructuring of Romania's state and private medicine has shaped people's responses to cervical cancer primary and secondary prevention programs.

PART 2 MEDICINE AND ITS MORALITIES

4 · DISMANTLING MEDICINE

> You want to know why I am not going to get a Pap test.... But you know
> what? Why would I go? What would happen to me if they found something
> wrong? What am I going to do then? Haven't you seen the wretched
> accommodation in the hospital?

Annoyed that I would wonder about her not taking advantage of free
cervical cancer screening, Adriana redirects the probing, her voice increasingly
more forceful with each new question to me. She has given me a tour of her vegetable garden and chicken coop and now we sit on her house veranda, drinking
Nescafé. A former unskilled factory worker, Adriana is unemployed, subsisting on
meager social benefits and paid manual labor that she does here and there for her
neighbors. At 48, she has recently become a grandmother. I joined her when she
visited her daughter and her newborn grandson at the local Roşiorii de Vede public hospital, and we both noticed the "wretched accommodation" to which she
alludes: worn-out furniture, dirty bed sheets, damp walls, foul smelling bathrooms.
Adriana pauses for a while, allowing me to fully grasp her exasperation, before adding in a lower, surrendering tone: "I don't even want to think about all this."

In Delcel district, other women shared Adriana's concerns about the quality
of public care. They would complain about the "wretched accommodation"
(*condiţiile mizere*) in state hospitals—a common trope in daily conversations.
But Adriana's outburst about the futility of getting a Pap smear was remarkable.
In previous chapters, I have recounted episodes from the reproductive life
histories of Oana, Ileana, Veturia, Maria, and others—most of them women in
their sixties and seventies—who had lived their reproductive years under communism. Their responses to the recently changing landscapes of sexual and
reproductive care originated in their past, often-traumatic experiences with
communist state medicine. Unlike the older women in the town, Adriana does
not situate her rebuttal of cervical cancer prevention in past traumas, historical
or personal. Rather, Adriana sees health as a future project, even if doomed to
failure. Her foot-dragging about the Pap test seems to be triggered by the difficulty of imagining a future whose uncertainties are rendered manifest by the
very idea of prevention.

As I came to realize, Adriana was voicing the views of many women who came of age in the late 1980s or even after 1989, whose stories I also recount in this book. Despite having relatively accurate knowledge about Pap tests and human papillomavirus (HPV) vaccines, women like Ana, Camelia, Călina, Ramona, and others in their twenties, thirties, and forties were ambivalent about cervical cancer prevention. Their reticence was not necessarily related to the accounts of their mothers, grandmothers, and other older women about reproductive vulnerability under communism. Their reserve was shaped by different historical circumstances. Adriana's outburst was remarkable because it made me realize that, to account for their perceived reproductive vulnerability, some women did more than just recount the past reproductive traumas they or others endured under communism. Her anxious questions were not as much directed at me as they were probing an ambiguous future. Like Adriana, other women also actively imagined their future reproductive health. In this chapter and those that follow, I address precisely this mutation from past quantifiable causes to future imagined possibilities, desires, and fears.

In this chapter, I continue exploring the systemic contingencies that have produced the cervical cancer crisis, and I highlight recent health care reforms as seen through the eyes of women from Roșiorii. In Romania, as elsewhere in the postcommunist world (Rivkin-Fish 2005; Andaya 2014; Ghodsee 2011; Brotherton 2012), the "dismantling of established legacies" (Bouzarovski, Sýkora, and Matoušek 2016, 628) has left many citizens disenfranchised. In response to state medicine reforms, people have used various tactics to access health care. These tactics—some old and repurposed, some new—both defy and welcome transformations to the medical system. I use the distinction between "strategy" and "tactic" to examine the impact of the strategic reforming of state medicine on Romanian women's tactics of accessing sexual and reproductive care. As de Certeau (2005, 220) has argued, "Lacking its own place, lacking a view of the whole, limited by the blindness (which may lead to perspicacity) resulting from combat at close quarters, limited by the possibilities of the moment, a tactic is determined by the *absence of power* just as a strategy is organized by the postulation of power."

In recounting women's raw, "blind," and tactical—rather than assertive and strategic—encounters with medical care in public hospitals, I show how they experience and conceptualize the mutations in state-subsidized medicine. I follow several women in their hypothetical rather than actual attempts to secure access to an OB-GYN specialist for a gynecological exam that may include a Pap test. Ana's story shows how mistrust in state medicine forced a mother to withhold her daughter from state-subsidized care all the way from conception and birth to the HPV vaccination. Ana's attitudes about state medicine and cervical cancer prevention were extreme. Other women had different opinions: Ramona appeared to endorse the HPV vaccine; Maria rejected the HPV vaccine despite her otherwise pro-vaccine attitude. Beyond the plurality of their views and experiences, women were, however, united in their deep mistrust in state medicine. Alongside women's accounts, I reflect on one of my own birthing experiences. Having a planned C-section in a public hospital turned out to be a time of intensive socialization into tactical engagements with medical workers and with the material conditions of care. While women's tactics are culturally and historically situated, Romanians are not unique in their rejection of the HPV vaccination. In the final part of this chapter, I briefly look at other controversial HPV vaccination campaigns worldwide and highlight the extent to which Romania's case illustrates the complicated and contradictory relationship between citizens and state governance.

Romanian women's tactics of navigating emerging regimes of care draw attention to their otherwise unintelligible responses to "free" prevention programs. As we shall see, while younger women's tactics of accessing (or rejecting) sexual and reproductive care are quite different from those of their mothers and grandmothers, there are intergenerational health-seeking behaviors that suggest important continuities in women's ideas about state medicine. Whether through the abuses of communist era pronatalism or confusing postcommunist reforms, state medicine has failed them all. Time and again, the state has proved to be either too much or not enough, as made painfully apparent through cervical cancer prevention programs. In the end, women's tactics provide us with yet another lens to understand the failure of state-driven cervical cancer prevention.

UPSIDE DOWN: REFORMING STATE MEDICINE

Ioana and her daughter-in-law, Ana, have invited me for a homemade cake tasting in their backyard. They live with Ioana's younger son—who is Ana's husband and the owner of a relatively prosperous small trucking company—and the couple's two pubescent children, a daughter and a son. Their house, one of the biggest in the whole neighborhood of Delcel, is a white-painted three-story villa with fake marble balcony railings. We sit around the table under a wax cherry tree, the July afternoon sun and the light breeze casting playful shadows through the branches onto the tablecloth. A retired baker, fifty-nine-year-old Ioana has continued to make custom cakes for clientele selected through word-of-mouth. Ana, whom I briefly introduced in chapter 2, is a twenty-nine-year-old housewife, and she occasionally helps her mother-in-law with her informal cake business.

Since I am visibly pregnant, the conversation quickly turns from patisserie to pregnancy, with Ioana proudly recalling how, more than thirty years ago, she was working long hours and even carrying flour sacks on her belly late into her pregnancies, to the disapproval of her OB-GYN. I ask Ioana and Ana about present-day pregnancy checkups; to my surprise, they disagree about the initial point of entry into prenatal care. While Ana asserts that a pregnant woman should go to the family doctor first, Ioana remembers self-referring directly to the gynecologist. A puzzled Ana turns to Ioana: "Why did you go to the gynecologist? You go to the family doctor, and *she* decides whether you should go further."

Thirty years between them, the dialogue between Ioana and Ana offered a glimpse into a generational shift in navigating reproductive care. Ana seemed to have little knowledge of pre-1989 polyclinic-based primary care. Until 1989, Romania's health care was state-owned and tax based, with universal coverage and free medical services for all. Primary care was provided at outpatient clinics—called polyclinics—by pediatricians, gynecologists, and generalists, and the medical system placed a strong emphasis on secondary and tertiary care (Grielen, Boerma, and Groenewegen 2000; Vlădescu et al. 2008). This is why the gynecologist was Ioana's point of entry into prenatal care. After 1989 and, more specifically, beginning in 1997, neoliberal-inspired reforms were introduced, aimed at an "unprecedented contraction in the size of the state" with drastically "decreasing government budgets" (Kutzin, Jakab, and Cashin 2010, 138). This led to a system of compulsory medical insurance through the establishment of the National Health Insurance Fund administrated by the National Health Insurance House (Casa Națională de Asigurări de Sănătate, or CNAS).[1] CNAS has contracts with both public and private health care providers (Vlădescu et al. 2008). Although still centralized, CNAS represents a transition from "implicit entitlements" to "explicit coverage" (Kutzin, Jakab, and Cashin 2010). In contrast with the past emphasis on secondary and tertiary care, the health care system has been reconceptualized "upside down" around the delivery of primary care by individually selected family physicians (*doctor de familie*).[2] Family physicians are also responsible for prenatal and postnatal visits, neonatal and infant care, and immunizations. The policy of refocusing on primary care has led to the closure of many rural dispensaries, polyclinics, and hospitals that once provided crucial health services to local populations (Bara et al. 2002).[3] As Ana emphasized, family doctors act as gatekeepers, so access to a specialist is contingent on their referral. But Ana's savvy coaching of her mother-in-law about the current referral system was ironic in more than one way. Such advice fell flat on Ioana. Like other women from Delcel who are past reproductive age, she understood menopause as granting one an exemption from any kind of gynecological checkups. It also turned out that Ana herself had never attended prenatal care during her pregnancies.

As in other Romanian towns of similar size, medical care is limited in Roșiorii. In 2013, the only public option for sexual and reproductive care was the OB-GYN section of the municipal hospital with three specialists. Two of them also worked in a private "medical center." Health Ministry organizational charts showed that, in 2015, the OB-GYN section of Roșiorii de Vede hospital was seriously understaffed, with only thirteen OB-GYN practitioners (doctors and nurses) of an estimated need of twenty, and six neonatal workers of a needed twenty.[4] By 2018, the hospital's obstetrics, gynecology, and neonatology resources had been further downsized as part of a restructuring that closed more than sixty-five OB-GYN units nationwide (Raț 2011). Victim to their proximity to Bucharest, medical personnel commute for work from Roșiorii to the capital city. As in other Romanian regional towns, in Roșiorii, this local mobility affects the fraction of health care workers who chose not to leave the country. But since 2002, and especially after 2007, massive waves of transnational professional emigrants left Romania, resulting in some of the sparsest territorial distribution of doctors, nurses, dentists, and pharmacists in Europe (Backman et al. 2008).[5] The medical brain drain prompted mass media to declare the entire Romanian medical system in a state of "clinical death." With mandatory rural internships for junior doctors discontinued, the few remaining medical workers are unevenly distributed and burned out by the long shifts necessary to cover frequent staff shortages. This was acknowledged in a February 2009 proposal to shorten the length of stay of doctors in maternity hospitals. Initiated by Ion Bazac, the health minister of the time, the proposal was a response to the tragic death of a mother from complications during birth in the maternity hospital of Comănești, a town in eastern Romania of a size comparable to Roșiorii de Vede. The woman had not been assisted at birth because the only OB-GYN specialist of the hospital had just left to go home, exhausted after completing a thirty-six-hour shift.[6]

Despite the "upside down" reconceptualization of state medicine, there are many continuities in people's experiences with public care. These are particularly visible in the practice of making informal payments to secure access to (privileged) forms of care. Referral procedures centered around the family doctor have perpetuated rather than discontinued the use of informal payments and connections, with patients making unsolicited under-the-table contributions to family physicians to secure access to certain specialists. I return to these practices in chapter 6, where I investigate women's informal contributions as tactics that redefine the moralities of reproductive care. For now, let us consider other tactics that women use to secure referrals or find a specialist, to navigate the material conditions surrounding health care delivery, to understand prevention, and to engage (or not) in preventive care.

SOMETHING OLD AND SOMETHING NEW

In responding to the changing landscapes of health care delivery, Romanians have mostly adapted old tactics of accessing care. Like Ana, other women from Delcel actively glossed over the new referral practices centered on the institution of the family doctor. Ramona, a forty-nine-year-old accountant, whose successful battle with infertility I described in chapter 1, compared her own experience of being pregnant in the 1980s with a hypothetical pregnancy under "the new system." Ramona started by recalling in detail monthly prenatal visits when the doctors routinely "checked" and "measured" her pregnant body in the polyclinic and later, when she started to experience complications, in the hospital. She added with a shrug: "Today you go to the family doctor and she refers you. It's a new system now." By condensing the description of the "new system" in one sentence, after giving an intricate account of the pre-1989 system, Ramona seems to imply that the quality of care in the past was better than in the present.

I asked women how they chose an OB-GYN specialist.[7] In some cases, they used online reviews to identify a doctor with a "good reputation." I had already noticed Delcel residents, including women in their fifties, sixties, and seventies, increasingly using the internet and online resources. Many of them were either divorced or widows whose adult children had relocated to Spain, Italy, or Germany; they had set up Skype and Facebook accounts to keep in touch with their children and grandchildren. Between Skype conversations, women navigated online in search of Orthodox pilgrimage bulletins, gardening advice, new recipes, and doctor reviews. The internet played a significant role in women's adoption of new tactics of access to care. Yet, although women sought input from a virtual community, most continued to rely, as in the past, on word-of-mouth: "The word spreads, that I gave birth with that one [doctor], and he is the best" (Tereza, age 57). "You have an acquaintance who tells you that he heard from another acquaintance that Doctor X treated Z and that he is a good man, too" (Andreea, age 25). Even women who used online reviews to find an OB-GYN specialist would usually test it against rumor and gossip and substantiate it by word-of-mouth. This may seem counterintuitive, but in marked continuity with previous tactics of access to medical care, information from established personal connections was paramount.

Most women referred to a generic family doctor using feminine forms of nouns and pronouns (*doctorița de familie*), but absolutely all used masculine forms of nouns and pronouns when talking about the OB-GYN specialist (*doctorul ginecolog*), despite increasing numbers of female OB-GYNs. In 2015, two out of the six OB-GYN specialists from Roșiorii de Vede municipal hospital were women. These linguistic cues reflect the degree to which patriarchy is embedded in reproductive care in contemporary Romania, a point that I illustrate further in chapter 5, when examining the gendered distinctions between public and private medicine made by Călina. After giving birth in a state hospital, Călina switched to a private one for her second birth. Călina's tactic of "birthing around" is new and atypical. The ethnographic data that I collected suggest that women from southern rural and peri-urban Romania continue practices of the past and do not routinely "shop around" for better care. Their tactics of finding a doctor are affected by predictable structural barriers such as lack of time, money, and transportation, but also by a sense of dutifully complying with a specialist's recommendations. While conceding that she had never experienced any serious health problems, Ana told me, with noticeable pride: "I never went to ask for a second opinion. I complied with what the first (doctor) told me to do. I never went to Bucharest for another set of laboratory analyses, and I never asked for another doctor's opinion, to challenge my doctor's." Overall, the prevalent ideal about an OB-GYN doctor is, as Andreea put it, of "a good man" who is said to be skillful. The tactics of actively relying on virtual information and personal communication to choose a doctor, and not really exploring alternatives that would challenge the doctor's authoritative (and quintessentially masculine) expertise, suggest a great deal of continuity in the way women conceptualize access to state reproductive medicine before and after 1989.

The continuities in women's tactical encounters with state medicine can also be observed in the way they engage with the actual provision of sexual and reproductive care. Giving birth in a public maternity hospital can challenge women to constantly readjust their sense of belonging and their ability to comply. The next three sections feature some of my own recollections of giving birth for the second time in a Romanian public maternity hospital.

PACKING THE HOSPITAL BAG

December 2009. I am sitting on the side of a cold and narrow surgery table in a public maternity hospital, very pregnant and completely naked, answering questions about my marital status and religious affiliation. My OB-GYN and his resident are standing by the table, their gloved hands up in the air, above their waistlines, waiting to start the C-section delivery. . . .

Earlier the same morning. I am thirty-eight weeks and four days pregnant. I wake up after a sleepless night and look through the window at the grim winter dawn. I am not in labor, but I know I will have my baby today because I am scheduled for a C-section delivery at one of the main public maternity hospitals of the city. I briefly go again through my hospital bag that I packed weeks ago: two nightgowns, a robe, underwear and socks, plastic slippers, a razor with a brand-new blade, towels, newborn diapers, baby wipes, diaper rash cream, a couple of pacifiers, onesies and other newborn apparel including scratch mittens, a small blanket, two packs of cotton wool, a breast pump, silicone nipple shields, nipple cream, cutlery, a plastic plate, a coffee mug, a large paper roll, toilet paper, books and magazines, notebook and pens, phone and charger, money in small bills, ID card (see figure 9). All is in place. I take a taxi to the hospital. I check in and am taken to a small, dilapidated waiting room, then instructed to change into the nightgown that I brought from home. No makeup and jewelry are allowed. Now I wait, alone, overwhelmed by anxious anticipation, shivering with cold in my thin nightgown. The hospital is under quarantine from swine flu, so access is restricted for the parturient women's relatives. Yet, I notice in the hallway a couple of fidgety fathers-to-be, and I realize that a small bribe to the doorman would probably have bent this interdiction. But I know that my baby's

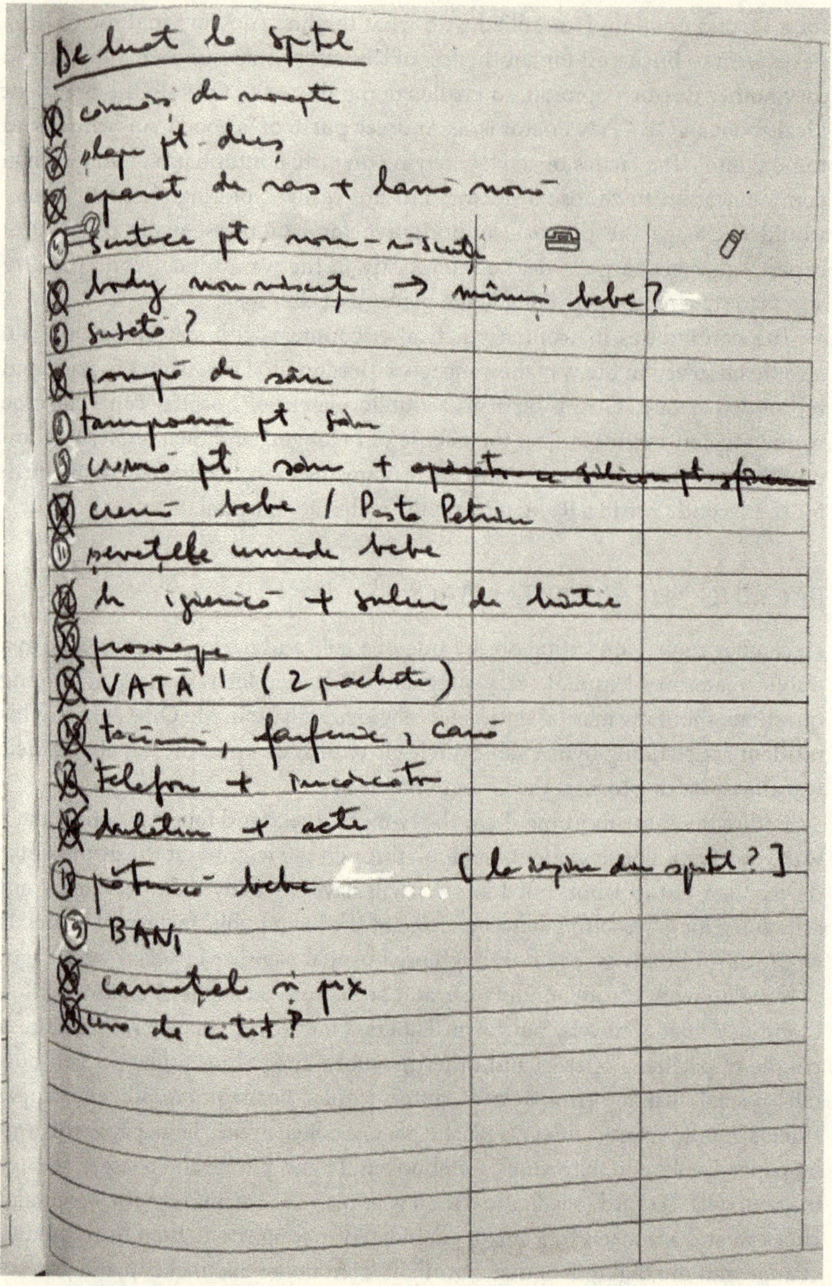

FIGURE 9. Hospital bag list made in preparation for my delivery in a public hospital in 2009. (Photo by the author.)

father had not planned to accompany me under any circumstance; he thinks that men don't belong in the birthing room. He is in a nearby café, anxiously sipping espressos.

COMPLIANCE, BOREDOM, HUMOR

Eventually, an edgy nurse enters the room. She cursorily inquires about my gestational age. She makes me sit on the consultation table and inserts an IV with normal saline into my left arm. She then pulls up the skirt of my nightgown with a sudden move that takes me by surprise and starts to scold me. I was supposed to have had my pubic hair removed before coming to the hospital. Humiliated but also vexed, I tell the nurse that I was only instructed by my OB-GYN to bring a razor with a brand-new blade, which I produce from my bag as proof of my compliance. Still grumbling, the nurse brings a small receptacle with cold water and soap and she skillfully shaves me. She then attaches a urinary catheter and opens almost completely the IV probe before leaving the room. The saline solution drips very fast; my left arm feels extremely cold. I sit and wait alone for half an hour. As instructed by the anesthesiologist, I had been fasting for eighteen hours and had had no liquid for twelve hours, and I am hungry and thirsty. Bored, I keep waiting. I look around me and try to imagine fantastic animal shapes in the old, cracked paint and the mold stains on the walls. I count the dirty floor tiles. I stare at the consultation table covered with a thick and cracked vinyl sheet of an unattractive shade of brown. The urinary catheter is uncomfortable, and my left arm is numb and frozen. The nurse returns to check and adjust the IV, which is now pouring the saline into my arm. I am placed in a wheelchair that the nurse pushes along hospital hallways to the surgical ward. The urinary catheter drainage bag hangs awkwardly between my legs, the IV probe is still inserted in my arm with the saline solution bottle sitting on my lap. When we reach the surgery unit, the nurse looks intently at me for the first time since we met, smiles, tells me that her shift is over and that I will be fine. She leaves with the empty wheelchair.

I look around the surgery theater. There is a high and narrow table in the middle, a huge powerful lamp above it, shockingly dirty PVC flooring, metallic shelves on a side with various medical instruments, an old issue of a tabloid newspaper. Next to the table I notice with some relief the friendly face of my OB-GYN, or at least that part of his face not covered with a mask. One of his residents and a nurse are also there. They all wear face masks, surgical scrub caps, gowns, and gloves. The doctor's cap features a funny and colorful cartoon design. They stand by the table with their hands up, above their waistlines, waiting to begin the C-section. I greet them. I walk slowly toward the table holding in my right hand the saline solution bottle that is still pouring through the IV in my left arm. I trip on the urinary catheter's drainage tube. Embarrassed, I joke about how, as an incorrigible fashionista, I follow the winter 2009 trends that highlight accessories such as IV tubes and urinary drains. We laugh, and the nurse helps me sit on the side of the table, my feet resting on a chair placed nearby. She pulls my nightgown up above my breasts, but the gown is too large and keeps falling back, so she removes it completely. I am naked, cold, and uncomfortable. The IV is removed from my arm. Yet, the delivery cannot start because the anesthesiologist is nowhere to be found. We wait in endless awkward silence. I am shaking of cold and emotion. Since the surgery is delayed, the nurse tries to keep me busy with filling a demographic profile form.

Finally, the anesthesiologist shows up and gives me the spinal shot. I am laid on my back and attached to the narrow table. A textile screen is placed above my waist to prevent me from seeing my lower body, numbed by the injection. The nurse is checking my vital signs through sensors attached to my chest and my fingers. After a few minutes, I hear a baby—my baby!—crying. Someone else—the neonatal doctor who had stepped in after the delivery began—places the newborn's warm cheek against mine and tells me, "You have a baby girl." She then takes the baby out of my sight. The doctor and his resident sew back the skin folds on my lower abdomen and exchange jokes with me. When they finish, they call for another nurse and for one of the hospital's doormen to help remove me from the table and carry me to the intensive care unit. There is no available stretcher and I am carried in their arms, wrapped in a thin sheet. At that moment I temporarily lose consciousness. . . .

TAMING THE HOSPITAL NIGHTSTAND

I wake up on a bumpy mattress in an intensive care unit (ICU) bed with spotty sheets. Someone had dressed me back in my nightgown. I touch my belly and discover yet another accessory—a drainage tube that comes out from the end of a long horizontal cut covered with a wide bandage. I already miss my baby, and I wonder not only where she is and how is she doing but what she looks like—I only got a cursory glimpse of her. I am told by an ICU nurse to not raise my head for the next six hours, until the effect of the anesthetic has worn off. So I am stuck to this bed, on my back, for the next six hours. All I can do is to move my head very slowly to the right and stare at the wall or to the left and contemplate a nightstand. I do the latter. It is a metal nightstand, a very common piece of furniture in most Romanian public hospitals. This one is painted all white, but I had seen others painted pale pink or faint blue. White or pastel—the paint is always chipped. With hours of forced immobility ahead of me, I contemplate the hospital nightstand and start to take mental field notes. This is a liminal object where ambiguities converge. It's a familiar piece of furniture that any patient would know from home, yet it appears foreign in a hospital setting. It divides a patient's vital space from that of the nearest roommate, but it also connects individual patients' personal spaces. It's functional, but its empty ugliness mobilizes patients and their family members to tame it. I recall the ritual of domesticating the hospital nightstand, opening the semi-stuck drawers and covering their rusty bottoms with wrapping paper or roll paper brought from home for this purpose. Once the drawer is padded, various personal items are placed inside: cutlery, plates, cosmetics, towels, the phone charger. Toilet paper. A few empty envelopes, in case "gifts" for medical staff take a monetary form. Then, the top of the nightstand also gets covered with roll paper, a decorative kitchen towel, or even a small macramé tablecloth, and on it, medication, a mug or a glass, a phone, books and magazines, pens, bottled water, and a vase with flowers. Sometimes, a small icon. By contemplating the hospital nightstand, a trained eye can decode a patient's diagnosis, the projected length of stay, maybe even the prognosis. . . .

My recollections above should be read as intimate descriptions of historically situated tactics of adjusting to the material conditions and human interactions that make possible a C-section in a public hospital from eastern Europe. The events that individualized my delivery also shaped similar reproductive experiences for the women of Roșiorii. During our conversations, we would occasionally reach moments of mutual recognition, when we acknowledged the shared value of our experiences with state reproductive medicine. As these recollections suggest, the material infrastructure and the interpersonal interactions that make possible a delivery in a public hospital shape the birthing experience for mothers, their families, and the medical staff. To ordinary people, these micro-interactions provide perhaps a more palpable sense of health care transformations than the macro-structural reforms. Some of the practices that other women, like me, engaged in accommodate change by linking past, present, and future. Packing the maternity bag and domesticating the hospital nightstand are tangible expressions not only of women's past experiences with state medicine but also of their current assumptions about the care they expect to receive. In the former communist countries of eastern Europe, patients and doctors routinely engage in "personalizing" tactics structured around the material contingencies of medical care. In a series of case studies, Michele Rivkin-Fish (2005) describes the unofficial gift exchanges between patients and medical workers in a maternity hospital from St. Petersburg, Russia. Similarly, Rima Praspaliauskiene (2016) retraces the under-the-table circulation of white envelopes with money that grant privileged care to patients in hospitals in Lithuania. I too was prepared to make informal payments. I did offer a monetary "gratitude gift" to the nurse who broke the rooming-in rule and took my daughter back to the neonatal ward for a few hours, after my initial failure to breastfeed left me exhausted. The actual tactics that people use are just a fraction of those they anticipate. Although I did not need to illicitly get any family member in the hospital, I was aware that bribing the doorman would have solved that problem. In addition to actively engaging with the material contingencies of health care, people may use what I call tactics of adequacy. These are meant to tame not the materiality of care but the specific temporality of care. In the clinical setting, boredom, humor, and navigating bureaucracy help patients fill a time that they cannot otherwise control. Finally, the wide array of tactics that people may employ serve not only to secure access to care or to successfully get through care. In some cases, women from Roşiorii mobilized their resources in order to avoid care altogether.

"IT IS NOT REQUIRED ANYMORE"

Irina has invited me into her newly renovated kitchen with ceramic tile floors, a running-water faucet, and a gas boiler—all innovations never seen before in her house. She ignored my request for tap water and instead, for both of us, poured Coca-Cola from a two-liter plastic bottle. I have to accept the sizzling soft drink—refusing it would only be perceived by my host as formal politeness. Irina was born in a small hamlet a few miles west of Roşiorii and commuted daily to town until she completed ten years of school. She married a factory foreman from Delcel, and they had two daughters together. At age 58, Irina had recently found herself *disponibilizată* ("released")—to use a term from the new wooden language of transition to market economy that sugarcoats the reality of unemployment—after the state-owned grocery where she worked for more than thirty years as an accountant was bought by a private company. After being forced into early retirement, Irina continued working as a freelancer bookkeeper for small local businesses.

While sipping our Coca-Cola, Irina responds to my question about the first thing women typically do after realizing they may be pregnant. They see a doctor, she tells me. When I continue asking her about pregnancy, Irina assures me, in an assertive tone, that pregnancy is a "normal state, not a disease." Irina gives me these answers—predictable from someone with high school education—in a quite automatic, default-like communication mode. To prompt her to actively reflect on the need for prenatal care, I point to the seeming paradox of seeing a doctor for a nonpathological "normal state." The purpose of an early prenatal exam, Irina responds, is to make sure that "everything is just fine" with both the expectant mother and the baby. By the end of my fieldwork in Delcel, I would have recorded this short conversational sequence repeated identically time and again with forty-three women. Of these women, forty-one answered without hesitation that, if she believed she was pregnant, a woman should see a doctor; all of them labeled pregnancy as "natural," "normal," "a given," "expected," or "common." Further prompted to justify a visit to a doctor for a "normal" condition, far from seeing any contradictions, women confidently emphasized the crucial role of the doctor in attesting to this state of normalcy.

These dialogues may suggest that women from Delcel were committed to a medicalized model of reproduction. However, despite their discursive endorsement of prenatal care, most of these women had not attended a gynecological or obstetrics examination for years and even for decades. Some women, Irina included, avoided as much as possible any prenatal and postnatal care, even when subjected to extreme reproductive surveillance, as occurred during the pronatalist era (1966–1989). Irina said she believed in prenatal care but confessed to avoiding it herself. How can we account for women's rhetorical commitment to reproductive medical care, yet their avoidance of it in practice? Irina's and others' discursive pledge to "see a doctor" may reflect their socialization into the system of "implicit entitlements" to care that were the foundation of pre-1989 universal coverage medicine. As Sean Brotherton (2012) explains, the emphasis of socialism in Cuba on medico-scientific progress and free access to health care has produced citizens with enhanced "medicalized subjectivities." Similarly, Romanians who grew up under communism were intensively exposed to the medicalization of life and health. Under pronatalism, the medicalization of pregnancy and birth took an extreme turn, as I described in chapters 1 and 2. More than just reproducing clichés about the value of medicine, Irina and many other women from Roşiorii want to be perceived as forward-looking modern women who are able to subscribe to biomedicine's contemporary discourses. After all, her new kitchen and Coca-Cola as her drink of choice literally showcased Irina's aspirations to align her lifestyle to that of western consumerist prosperity.

Enthusiastic discourses aside, only two of the forty-three women acknowledged having had a Pap smear in the past ten years. Another twenty-seven were unsure whether they had ever had the test, although most provided an accurate description of it. Finally, as I mentioned in chapter 3, fourteen women—all over forty-five years old—claimed that they had never heard of the test, although all had some knowledge of cervical cancer and knew that it could be detected at early stages. Despite their diverse experiences with cervical cancer secondary prevention in the form of the Pap test, most women did not prioritize preventive gynecological controls. Significantly, the women who did not know about the Pap smear were more likely than their counterparts to see preventive gynecological controls in historical rather than biomedical terms. They considered the post-1989 termination of the mandatory gynecological exams the most important recent transformation in sexual and reproductive care. In a group discussion, Ramona (age 49) explained: "Before [1989], you would go to the doctor and he would report that you were there, for the control. They don't have to report nowadays." Ileana (age 59) concurred: "Before [1989] you had to go to the gynecological control. During communism they suspected that you concealed a pregnancy if you didn't go. Today nobody watches," while Adriana (age 48) concluded: "Now, each [woman] chooses whether to go or not [to a gynecological control]." Like some of her peers, Irina also associates preventive reproductive care with the past, both historical and personal: "I haven't had a gynecological exam since the birth of my younger daughter, twenty-eight years ago. Before

[1989] it was different. During Ceauşescu's time, women had to go to the dispensary for medical checkups all the time."

Irina, however, has avoided gynecological exams not only because they encapsulate something about the state's past political surveillance. She also points to her partner's uneasiness about her naked body being exposed for medical scrutiny: "My husband was upset about all these exams, and I didn't like it either . . . undressing in front of the doctor, with the nurses, with all those people around. But nowadays nobody cares about [gynecological] controls."

Irina then continues her account about gynecological exam avoidance, confiding: "I am getting older, I am not much of a woman anymore . . . but I feel good, I am still strong." First, Irina reiterated major themes that I explored in previous chapters, from the biopolitical surveillance of female reproductive bodies to the persistence of patriarchal forms of control over women's sexuality and reproduction. Like Ramona and Ileana, Irina explicitly contrasted the two regimes of reproductive health care delivery—the mandatory pronatalist controls of the communist era versus the voluntary medical exams of present-day. Second, she recalled gynecological exams as embarrassing episodes, a reaction amplified by her husband's disapproval of her being subjected to intimate medical consultations (see also Grigore et al. 2017). In rural areas, cervical cancer is more highly stigmatized than other cancers (Todorova et al. 2006) because it affects the "shameful parts" (părțile rușinoase)—that is, women's genitals. Some of the women from Delcel confessed that their reluctance to get a gynecological exam was in part amplified by the commonly held belief that only promiscuous women would acquire sexually transmitted infections. Third, Irina's elusive reference to menopause hinted at the patriarchal understanding of womanhood as defined by reproductive promise. As Irina put it, a menopausal woman was "not much of a woman anymore." In the end, Irina fashioned a personal statement about the futility of preventive reproductive medicine by weaving together her own traumatic recollections of the pronatalist regime and her (and her husband's) patriarchal understandings of a woman's body and sexuality.

Irina was not unique in her decades-long avoidance of reproductive care. Twenty other women who confessed to not having had a gynecological exam since 1989 rationalized this by contrasting past and present regimes of reproductive medicine. "I haven't seen a gynecologist since 1989. It is not required [to do so] anymore"—I would keep hearing them say during our conversations. Women's avoidance of (preventive) reproductive care may seem unintelligible, especially when considered in light of the neoliberal-inspired medical reforms that presume patients-turned-consumers' active pursuit of health and well-being. We can ask, however, whether normative expectations about women constantly engaging in gynecological exams would not amount, again, to an essentialization of women as reproducers (Inhorn 2006). After all, as Lock and Kaufert noted, "For most women, reproduction does not occupy an undue proportion of their energy"

(1998, 19). Tactical avoidance of gynecological controls may, in fact, be a way to exert agency in the form of low-key resistance aimed at the "pragmatic rather than ideological" reappropriation of their own bodies (Lock and Kaufert 1998, 11; Scott 1985). The notion of resistance seems to be central to understanding why women might refuse to see a gynecologist. Statements such as "it is not required [to see a gynecologist] anymore" emphasize the power of individual choice to gloss over the (un)availability of official resources. After decades of state paternalism, many women deliberately use avoidance as an empowering tactic, even if, in the end, it may have consequences on their health.

Resistance to gynecological exams, Pap tests, and HPV vaccination cannot be detached from Romanians' fraught relationship with the state. In light of their experiences with communist reproductive medicine, women perceive the state almost oxymoronically as the coercive provider of care. Together with their rhetorical commitment to biomedicine, women's avoidance of preventive reproductive care reveals both an aspiration to benefit from medical care entitlements and a need to resist official channels of health care delivery. Women's ambivalence proves that far from being passive recipients, they actively work around biomedicine's values, discourses, and resources. Talking about the HPV vaccine, Adriana actively interrogated these landscapes of uncertainty: "On the one hand, I would say [the vaccine] is a good thing, but on the other, I heard that it is not good; it can make you sicker. I don't know what the best thing would be [to get the vaccine or not]. What would be the right thing to do?"

"It is not required anymore" is more than a simple acknowledgment of shifting regimes of health care delivery. The avoidance of gynecological exams captures something from ordinary women's mistrust in both past state medicine and in its contemporary version. While reproductive surveillance ended, adequate reproductive care has only been provided inconsistently in a country marred by a difficult postcommunist transition. Ileana's comment that "today nobody watches" (*nimeni nu se uită*) can be understood in more than one way: She may refer to surveillance ("watches you"), care ("watches over you"), or maybe both. Indirectly, these women cast blame both on the communist state's centralized paternalism and on the postcommunist state's centrifugal fragility. As Ana's story illustrates below, by withholding their daughters from the HPV vaccine, parents challenged the legitimacy of a type of governance that they perceived as intrusive but uncaring. Despite recent shifts in regimes of health care delivery, these women saw health as a state-controlled project.

REPRODUCTION ON THE MARGINS

Ioana's daughter-in-law, Ana, is the mother of a twelve-year-old girl and nine-year-old boy. I ask Ana about her decision not to allow her daughter to receive the HPV vaccine. Before answering, Ana detours to describe in detail her daughter's birth. During her first pregnancy, she was a teenager and a high school student. Since she was under eighteen, she could not legally marry the child's father but lived with him at her future parents-in-law's house. Ana did not have a pregnancy checkup because she "was feeling just fine," and although she suffered what she calls "a calcium meltdown" (*cădere de calciu*) and temporary facial hemiparesis (*semipareză*), she did not see a doctor. Neither her mother nor her mother-in-law advised Ana to see an obstetrician, because the mandatory reporting of pregnancies had been discontinued after 1989. Like other women from Delcel, Ana alludes to the end of pronatalist policies enforced during Ceaușescu era, and although she was only nine years old in 1989, it shows again the power of oral histories to shape the attitudes of the younger generations.

Ana gave birth to a premature baby girl at about thirty weeks gestation, healthy but weighing only 1,700 grams (3.7 pounds). Although the local municipal hospital of Roșiorii de Vede, where she gave birth, was under strict policy not to release the mother and the infant until the baby's weight reached 2,500 grams (5.5 pounds), Ana pretended to have "an attack of hysteria crisis" so that she was permitted to take the baby home immediately. Sobbing, she explained to the medical staff: "I want [to go] home, because there my mom-in-law will supervise me. Women who know [about caring for babies] will supervise me." Ana is obviously proud of having skipped both prenatal and postnatal institutionalized care. She leans toward me and raises her eyebrows: "Ask me when I *first* went to the hospital!" Excited to read the anticipated perplexity on my face, Ana exclaims: "When I gave birth! I gave birth and I came home." With the help of Ioana, her mother-in-law, and Crina, her sister-in-law, Ana managed to take good care of her premature daughter and breastfed for nineteen months. Looking intently at me, Ana proclaims: "Maternal milk was the healthiest for the baby." Caught up in this birth story, I wonder for a moment how we ended up talking about breast milk when I had asked Ana about refusing the HPV vaccine for her daughter.

But Ana makes a point. In recalling her pregnancy, childbirth, and lengthy breastfeeding experience, she claims that, from conception, she has kept her daughter away from official medical practices. That Ana's avoidance of professional medical care was more than a teenager's recklessness was proved when, twelve years later, her daughter was in the target population for the HPV vaccination. Ana refused. Pointing presumably in the direction of her daughter's room, Ana continues with growing frustration, contrasting her daughter's actual well-being and innocence to the alleged health benefits: "Look at her: She's just fine, and she's only a child. They vaccinate her *just in case* . . . and if she would not be vaccinated and *the case* would happen, so what? Since they managed to make a vaccine, they should try to come up also with a treatment, or a medicine or something, to take only if you get sick [in order to] to recover."

Ana's birthing story of no prenatal care and minimal postnatal supervision, on the margins of medicalization, is not necessarily atypical in peri-urban and rural Romania. While most women with whom I spoke were rather skeptical of the HPV vaccine and the Pap test, not all were as determined as Ana to shield themselves and their daughters from cervical cancer prevention. The most notable exception was Ramona, who seemed to openly embrace the HPV vaccination.

OTHER VOICES, SAME MISTRUST

It is a hot August afternoon. Ramona and I sit in the living room of her top-floor apartment in a concrete apartment building of the late communist era. Cold and damp in winter, the poorly insulated building is a suffocating oven in summer. The living room has a balcony whose door, although open, does not let in any fresh air. Like her neighbors, Ramona and her husband sealed their balcony to insulate their place from the winter's cold biting winds. But in August, the balcony is a veritable greenhouse, adding to the living room heat. The apartment smells strongly of roasted eggplant. To my joy, Ramona brings into the living room a bowl of freshly made, still warm eggplant salad and a few slices of crispy bread. Ramona is keen and confident. A college graduate, she works for a large private business in Roşiorii, receiving a monthly salary that secures her a comfortable living by local standards.[8] Ramona's job duties include frequent trips to Bucharest, and she repeatedly boasts about her cosmopolitan mobility. At forty-nine, she has been married for thirty years to her college sweetheart, a construction engineer. I look around the room at family pictures. Ramona is very proud of the professional achievements of her only child, a daughter she had after an extended period of infertility, as described in chapter 1. After graduating from the medical school in Bucharest, Ramona's daughter relocated to the United Kingdom, where she works as a doctor.

We have been talking about reproductive health care, and I ask Ramona about her opinion on the HPV vaccination campaign. To my surprise, Ramona's voice changes. She explains, suddenly struggling to find her words: "If [the Health Ministry] decided to organize the HPV campaign... and I don't think they decided... I think it is good." Mistaking Ramona's sudden faltering for a clue that my question may have been too open-ended, I ask her to imagine a concrete situation. Were her daughter younger, would she consent to her vaccination? Visibly uncomfortable, fidgeting, and avoiding looking directly at me, Ramona gives me an oblique answer: "Since a campaign is going on, I think it is good to be vaccinated at any time." I remind her that the vaccine is presumably more effective if given before starting sexual life.[9] Nervously rewinding her wristwatch, Ramona bursts into a high-pitch tirade:

No, it is not possible to control people's sexual activity. You can have [sexually active] girls as young as thirteen years old. I think that is the right way [to vaccinate]. I believe that they wouldn't decide this without knowing that it was good.

Some studies must have been made, some research.... We are not anymore in the eighteenth century to do experiments on humans, and at this scale ... at a national scale?

As I listened to the recorded interview and reviewed my notes during transcription, I was struck by the change in Ramona's attitude when we tackled the HPV vaccine issue. Her voice was higher, she was more hesitant, she paused more often and did not finish some of her sentences ("If they have decided this ... I don't think they decided this just for ..."). Even when she made a confident statement ("I think this is the right way"), Ramona switched immediately to an unsolicited explanation about the presumed scientific evidence ("some studies must have been made, some research") that was vague enough to weaken her position. She continued with a few rhetorical questions that seemed to challenge an invisible opponent, perhaps the result of opinions she had heard from others ("experiments on humans, and at this scale ... at a national scale?"). While she appeared to endorse the vaccine, Ramona was somehow uncomfortable with the topic, as suggested by her use of discourse markers such as pausing, using a high-pitch voice, providing oblique answers, and raising rhetorical questions. She also avoided directly answering my hypothetical question about her daughter being vaccinated. Like Irina and others, Ramona's commitment to biomedicine was more rhetoric than real.

Although atypical compared to other women and their resistance to cervical cancer prevention, Ramona's words provide a glimpse into the popular reactions to the HPV vaccination campaign. As I explore further in chapter 6, most people I spoke with expressed suspicion about the official public health justification of the HPV campaign. Ramona was willing to trust the government to some extent, but she could not completely ignore a history of terrible past experiments conducted in the name of science and progress. In the end, she struggled to reconcile competing discourses of modernity—one that recognizes the benefits of a quintessential biomedical procedure like vaccination, and the other that delegitimizes the state on the grounds of its maximal intrusion into women's health and well-being.

Maria, the seventy-four-year-old woman featured in chapters 2 and 3, also had a distinct reaction to my questions about the HPV vaccination. I helped her carry inside her house a few wooden logs for her stove, and we resumed the conversation, while sitting on her porch. Tilting her head left and right, as if in doubt, Maria asks me: "Do you really want to get that [HPV] vaccine?" Rather than rejecting the HPV vaccine, Maria seems willing to discuss it, even though her question appears to be rhetorical. Then, she continues, rolling up her sleeve and showing me a white wrinkled spot on her sunburned arm: "The real vaccine is the one that you receive here, in your arm." The mark on her arm is from the Bacille Calmette-Guerin (BCG) vaccine, a tuberculosis (TB) vaccine routinely given to newborns in Romania since 1926. Given that the Romanian health authorities introduced all the other infant immunizations from the early 1960s, when Maria was already an adult, the BCG vaccine is probably the only vaccine that she ever received. By calling the BCG "the real vaccine," she attempted to delegitimize the HPV vaccine. Maria elaborated: "Now you go with the child to be pricked and misfortunes happen. This is not normal. It may protect you, but have you seen how many problems have occurred with the vaccine?" As Maria framed it, the contrast between the "real" vaccine and the HPV vaccine reflected a temporal opposition between a resourceful past and contested present, routine and exception, order and chaos. Her questioning of the HPV vaccine incapsulated a critique of the present-day state medicine. Extrapolating from controversies about the HPV vaccination campaign as reported on TV, Maria—like others, as I show in chapter 6—imagined an unsettling world of serial "misfortunes." When she proudly showed me the TB mark on her arm, she conveyed to me in a palpable way that she had benefited from a successful vaccination under a systematic and predictable regime of health care delivery. By contrast, in the present-day, with the HPV vaccine "pricked" instead of "injected"—she emphasized the intrusive and unpredictable character of medical care. Maria was not atypical of people who acknowledged (and were proud of) being vaccinated yet did not endorse the HPV vaccination campaign. Romanians did not really resist other vaccines in the past, and this makes the HPV controversy even more remarkable. However, resistance to the HPV vaccine may have created a precedent, by bringing into visibility vaccination anxieties more generally. For instance, acceptance rates of the measles-mumps-rubella (MMR) vaccine have declined in Romania in the past ten years, especially among urban Orthodox and educated parents (Pop n.d).

Some other women, like forty-three-year-old Ilinca, were more adamant in their rejection of the HPV vaccine: "I am not going to let my daughter be vaccinated! Stop forcing us to swallow (*nu ne mai băgaţi pe gât*) what others decide [for us]!" Similarly, fifty-year-old Paula told me: "Do you know why there are so many polemics about the HPV vaccine? Because this is the way people react when they are forced to swallow new things." On several occasions, other people voiced their anxieties about the HPV vaccination through idioms of forced feeding. Ilinca, Paula, and others used "swallowing" as a metaphor for acquiescence (Lakoff and Johnson [1980] 2003). By refusing to swallow the HPV vaccine they did not acquiesce to the legitimacy of the state controlling young bodies. The forced-feeding idioms also hinted at ways by which vaccination violated the integrity of bodily boundaries. Like the pricking metaphor that Maria used to refer to the injection, forcing someone to swallow something transforms the person into a powerless recipient. With vaccination, bodies are made into passive entities into which medication is "forced" through subcutaneous injection. As we shall see next, questioning the HPV vaccination is part of a broader attitude of contestation of the state legitimacy to mandate preventive care.

THE STATE OF VACCINES: TOO MUCH, YET NOT ENOUGH

One Sunday evening, as we stroll around the neighborhood, thirty-eight-year-old Gabriela, a supermarket clerk, tells me in a bitter voice: "[There are] too many cases of mothers dying in childbirth. . . ." In the peaceful lilac-smelling dusk of May, her words take me by surprise. Here and there, people sit on benches on the sidewalk, smoking and chatting and greeting us, as we walk by. The occasional dog bark only makes the silence of the evening even deeper. Perched on an electricity pole, three storks are quietly fixing their nest. But Gabriela continues with earnest frustration: "I mean, they used to give birth in the house wagon, on the fields, poor things, and you didn't hear about them dying in childbirth. And now, all you hear on TV is that mothers die in childbirth, in a hospital, with doctors, with specialists." Like Maria, who did not question the old TB vaccine mark on her arm but critically scrutinized the new HPV vaccine, Gabriela also romanticizes past regimes of reproduction while she emphasizes the failure of present-day medicine to care for the most vulnerable—pregnant women and their babies. The world of vulnerability that she describes is one in which reproduction is problematic. It's an "unnatural" world in which death substitutes life. After the fall of the communist regimes in eastern Europe, the state lost its grip as a "strong mediating force" on the "relationship between 'the individual' and the socially constructed 'natural' order" (Kaneff 2002, 97). People started to question the role of the government and the structures of governance in unprecedented ways. Romanians' resistance to the national HPV vaccination campaign occurs in the context in which state legitimacy came under scrutiny with the end of the communist era.

The HPV vaccination sits at the intersection of two of the most contested forms of state governance: vaccination and reproductive policies. Part of biomedicine's project of standardizing local biologies, vaccination was made into an effective biopolitical tool when regulated by state authorities into national immunization programs (Lock and Nguyen 2010; Connell and Hunt 2010). Vaccination campaigns such as the anti-tetanus vaccination in Cameroon (Feldman-Savelsberg, Ndonko, and Schmidt-Ehry 2000) and Mozambique (Chapman 2010), the anti-polio vaccination in Niger (Masquelier 2012) and Nigeria (Renne 2010), and the measles and rubella immunization in Ukraine (Bazylevych 2011) have provided anthropologists with opportunities to document people's complicated reactions. In these accounts, vaccination compliance or refusal are seen as "local responses to global and/or national projects" (Feldman-Savelsberg, Ndonko, and Schmidt-Ehry 2000). Accepting a vaccine can indicate "confidence in the safety and efficacy of that particular technology and trust in the public health system to deliver the technology safely" (Kaufman 2010, 19). Conversely, vaccination campaigns have generated intense contestation of the state's (mis)management of health care. Rada, a thirty-six-year-old mother of one baby girl, opined: "I think that this vaccine does more harm than good. The vaccination campaign is like other [campaigns] undertaken by the Ministry, just a source of income for the pharmaceutical industry. Nothing good for our girls." Monica, twenty-nine, added: "The vaccination campaign is salutary, but it is also confusing. It is a controversial vaccine. I would not have my girl inoculated, were she old enough."

Romania's unsuccessful HPV vaccination campaign was not an isolated case. Proposals to vaccinate girls against HPV generated heated political, ethical, and public health controversies in several countries, including in huge drug markets such as the United States and India. In these countries, HPV vaccination triggered concerns about the state mandate to control young women's reproductive health.[10] However, such anxieties have had a particular poignancy in Romania in the light of past and present state reproductive policies. Aura, a forty-year-old family doctor, was blunt in her assessment of the HPV vaccination campaign: "You don't want to play Russian roulette with your daughter just for the sake of the Health Ministry." As Irina, Ramona, Ileana, and others admitted, after more than forty years of communist paternalism, people's reflexes regarding state control over women's reproductive health are inherently contradictory. Many women felt entitled to free reproductive care in public hospitals, but, like Gabriela, they expressed frustration at the state's failure to provide adequate care. On the one hand, they expected to be taken care of by a resourceful state; on the other hand, they blamed the controlling state for intruding into their private lives.

CONCLUSIONS

In the aftermath of the communist regime's demise, Romanians have responded to the changing landscapes of state reproductive medicine in a tactical rather than strategic manner. Some of the tactics of accessing and securing adequate care, as I described in this chapter, reveal remarkable continuities with everyday practices from the communist era. Ethnography allows us to highlight these continuities that occur despite the dismantling of the old medical system (see also Ghodsee 2011). Women's tactical responses to reproductive care as delivered by the state both capitalize on and expose citizens' mistrust in state medicine. Situated at the intersection of reproduction and vaccination—both sites of cultural and political contestation—the HPV vaccination campaign worked to expose the ambiguities of postcommunist governance. To the women from Delcel, from the vantage point of national cervical cancer prevention, the state appears at the same time excessive and weak. As I illustrate it in chapter 5, the confusion around cervical cancer prevention created by public care reforms only deepened with the emergence of private reproductive medicine, with its (dis)similar networks of care.

INTERLUDE
Cervical Cancer Prevention: A Romanian Odyssey (Part 2)

On March 19, 2013, Mihaela Geoană, the president of Renașterea Foundation, a nongovernmental organization (NGO), made a special guest appearance on a live show on *Antena 3* TV to discuss human papillomavirus (HPV) vaccination. Geoană blamed Romania's exceptionally high cervical cancer mortality on women's reluctance to seek preventive sexual and reproductive care. When she asserted that "prevention starts with HPV vaccination," an uppercase caption at the bottom of the TV screen read: "THE DIFFERENCE BETWEEN LIFE AND DEATH: THE VACCINE" (*Diferența între viață și moarte: vaccinul*) (figure 10).

Geoană's interview is worth our attention for several reasons. First and perhaps most importantly, construing the HPV vaccine as the life-bearing variable in a generic life-or-death case marked an unprecedented radicalization of the promotion of HPV vaccination in Romania. Geoană and the advertisers behind her assumed that simply opposing life to death would intuitively speak to everyone. As long as the vaccine represented life, vaccination would be the obvious choice. However, as I show in this book, Renașterea's generic and nonproblematic life-or-death HPV vaccination promotion missed the mark by ignoring the complex and systemic contingencies of living and dying as a woman in present-day Romania.

Second, the show featured the president of Renașterea herself. The foundation was created in 2001 as an NGO for "education, health, and culture." Seven years later, the government granted the foundation the status of public interest organization. Renașterea was then rebranded as "a foundation for women's health." As Renașterea's president, Geoană spoke neither as a state representative nor as a private profit maker. She only claimed to represent women's best interest. That the intended power of Geoană's message originated in her politically nonaffiliate position is significant, given the government corruption allegations that surrounded the HPV vaccination campaign. However, Geoană's position was not perceived as neutral by most people, and her foundation came under

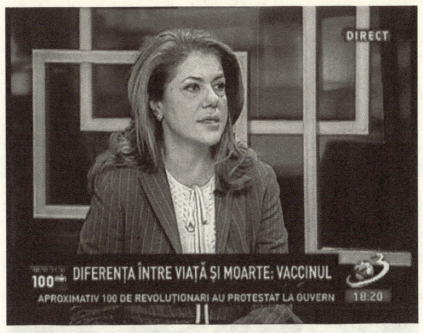

FIGURE 10. Still frame from Geoană's live interview on *Antena 3*.

public scrutiny for presumed conflicts of interest and illicit associations with both state executives and private pharmaceutical companies. This was in part because Geoană's husband is a prominent political figure in Romania. A career diplomat, Mircea Geoană served as the Romanian ambassador to the United States. He was later the Minister of Foreign Affairs, the social-democrat presidential candidate in the 2009 elections, and the president of the Senate.

Third, Geoană is neither a medical nor a pharmaceutical professional. Whether in Romania or elsewhere, the HPV vaccination debates involved, maybe more than for any other vaccine, a sheer number of nonexperts, from journalists, politicians, and political analysts to members of the clergy, bloggers, and conspiracy theorists. Furthermore, as I mentioned in the first interlude, when a well-established epidemiologist like Dr. Streinu-Cercel endorsed the vaccine, his professional expertise was overshadowed by public accusations regarding his moral standing.

Finally, Geoană's televised intervention raised awareness about the role that NGOs played as alternatives to state-controlled channels of cervical cancer preventive care delivery. In response to the stalling of the official HPV vaccination campaign, more than a year before Geoană's interview, in November 2011, several professional organizations and NGOs had created a Coalition for Cervical Cancer Prevention (CCCP). This coalition included Renașterea Foundation, the Society of Obstetrics and Gynecology, the Pediatric Society, and the National Society for Family Medicine. On January 24, 2012, during the European Week

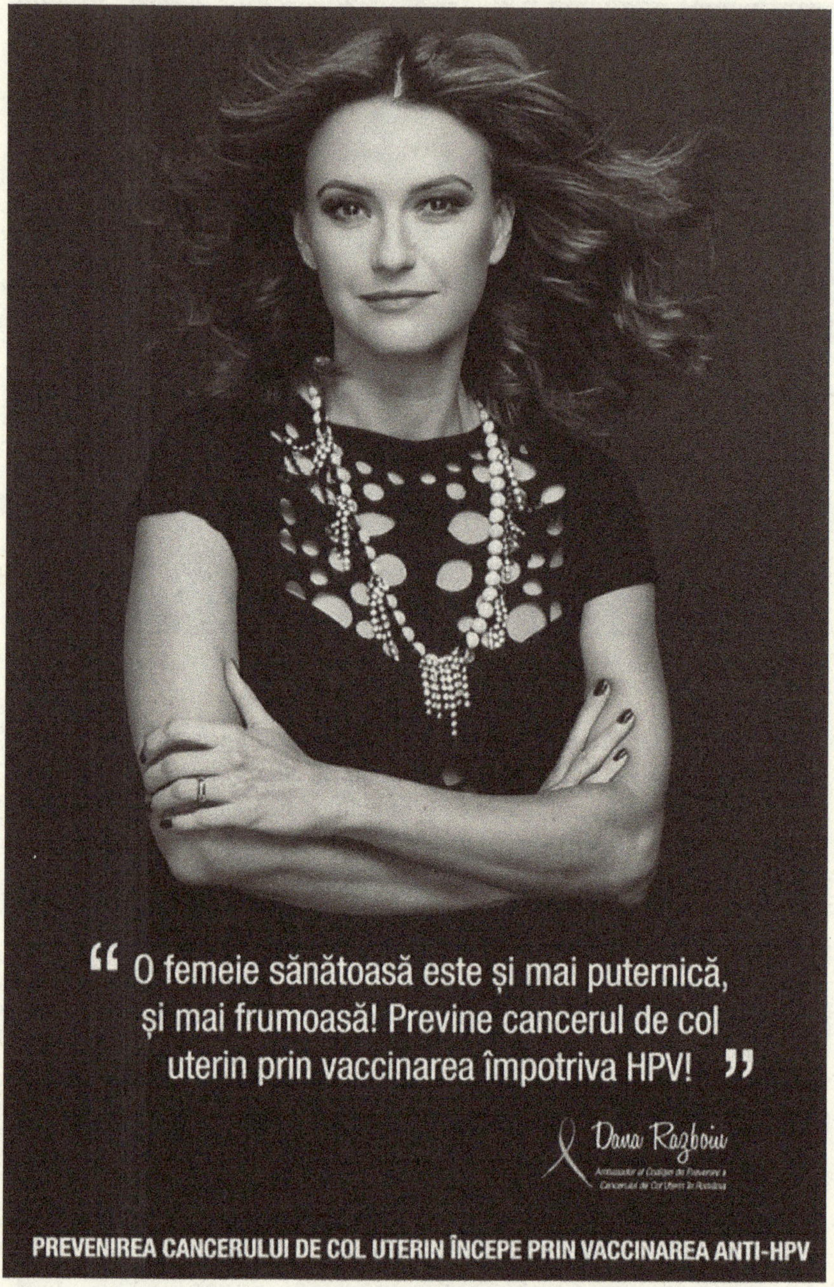

> ❝ O femeie sănătoasă este și mai puternică, și mai frumoasă! Previne cancerul de col uterin prin vaccinarea împotriva HPV! ❞

Dana Razboiu
Ambassador of Coaliția de Prevenire a
Cancerul de Col Uterin în România

PREVENIREA CANCERULUI DE COL UTERIN ÎNCEPE PRIN VACCINAREA ANTI-HPV

FIGURE 11. Missing the mark: women and girls from Delcel (on the right, photo by the author) did not recognize themselves in the cervical cancer prevention ideal of health and beauty represented by Războiu (on the left). (Source: https://www.facebook.com /CervicalCancerPreventionRomania/.)

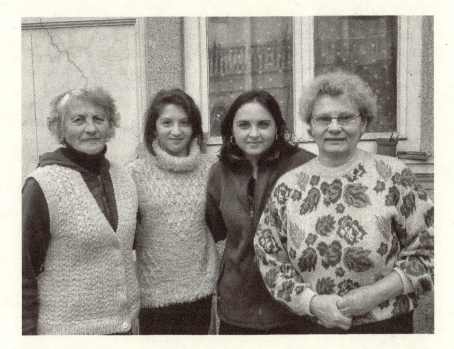

for Cervical Cancer Prevention, Renașterea organized a press conference, releasing the report "Romania Ranks High: Cervical Cancer Strikes Again." The document's headlines read: "Cervical cancer is easy to detect. Every day, six women die of cervical cancer in Romania. Field data showed that about 70 percent of the women enrolled in a study had complex genital infections." During the press conference, Renașterea representatives advertised their mobile clinic screening program for women in underserved areas. The program had reportedly detected high rates of sexually transmitted infections (STIs) and of abortions used as a method for fertility control. During the 2012 European Week for Vaccination, CCCP organized a roundtable on the HPV vaccine, hosted by the U.S. Embassy in Bucharest. The event featured the U.S. ambassador, Renașterea Foundation representatives, and epidemiologist Streinu-Cercel.

Despite the stalling of the state-driven campaign, the coalition continued to promote the HPV vaccine until 2015, when it stopped updating its Facebook page. For the 2013 European Week for Cervical Cancer Prevention, the coalition set up a vaccination awareness campaign that featured telegenic journalist Dana Războiu as the "ambassador" for the Coalition for Cervical Cancer Prevention. The CCCP posters urged young women to "prevent cervical cancer by getting the HPV vaccine" (*Previne cancerul de col uterin prin vacinarea HPV!*). Wearing perfect makeup and extravagant oversized jewelry, Dana Războiu looked boldly into the camera lens (figure 11). The two versions of the poster included, between quotation marks, Războiu's opinion about the vaccine enabling health as a personal project ("A healthy woman is stronger and more beautiful!" [*O femeie sănătoasă este și mai puternică și mai frumoasă!*]) and health as a responsibility ("The most important thing for your family is to take care of your own health" [*Cel mai important lucru pentru familia ta este să ai grijă de sănătatea ta!*]).

CCCP also designed a template document intended for use by parents who had decided to ask their family doctors to administer the HPV vaccination to their daughters. Independent from the Coalition for Cervical Cancer Prevention, which appeared to be inactive after 2015, the NGO Renașterea continued to organize annual events promoting cervical cancer prevention, every January between 2016 and 2020. However, the campaigns have become more and more basic, with broad, generic slogans such as "Stop cervical cancer!" used in 2016 and again in 2019. If the government-managed HPV vaccination has undergone a dramatic downsizing over the years, with decreased vaccine supply distribution, the NGO-driven cervical cancer awareness and prevention has not fared better, either. With recycled promotion materials and lingering social media pages, cervical cancer prevention has dwindled. As of 2021, it appears that what has been stopped is not cervical cancer but governmental and nongovernmental cervical cancer prevention programs.

5 · THE OTHER HOSPITAL

November 2009. Thirty-four weeks into my pregnancy, I wake up with mild contractions. I call my OB-GYN, who has been following my pregnancy at his private practice. He tells me to come for an emergency consultation to the public teaching hospital where he is full-time affiliated as an assistant professor of obstetrics and gynecology at the medical school. I wait in the hallway, chatting with another pregnant woman who is here to see the same doctor. She turns out to be not quite an ordinary patient. She introduces herself as Doctor MT, a gynecologist in a small town of northern Romania. I tell her that I am a medical anthropologist, and our chat turns into an ad hoc interview about the pros and cons of giving birth in an underresourced public hospital in a city with available private care alternatives. Both Doctor MT and I believe that only the best professionals secure positions in university hospitals. We perceive our OB-GYN as more qualified than most doctors affiliated with the private clinics. Although there are at least two public and two private maternity clinics in the city, Doctor MT and I refer in our conversation to a generic private maternity hospital as "the other hospital" (*celălalt spital*). We both express the—empirically unsubstantiated—conviction that "the other hospital" has less prestigious and less experienced doctors. Yet, giving birth in this hospital is not only about the professional reputation of its medical staff. As Doctor MT explains, only state maternity hospitals are able to manage premature births and unforeseen neonatal complications. Private clinics do not provide neonatal intensive care.[1] As an OB-GYN herself, Doctor MT's thinking is shaped more than mine by the idea of perinatal risk. We thus agree, while fidgeting on the uncomfortable chairs of the waiting area, that "the other hospital" is riskier for both parturient mothers and their newborns.

Following this impromptu hallway discussion, I feel really good about my decision to give birth for the second time in a public hospital, despite the fact that two private clinics had opened in town since my first birth. Still absorbed in these self-congratulatory thoughts, I am finally let into a decrepit examination room. Nothing seems to have improved since the last time I gave birth in this hospital, almost three years earlier. Insidiously, the shiny ghost of "the other hospital" comes haunting me. I cannot help but think about the presumably much better patient accommodation and medical technology of private clinics. The consultation room is, to my surprise, very crowded. It is clinical practice day for my OB-GYN's students. As I lie on my back on the gynecological table, naked from my waist down with no gown provided by the hospital, two medical residents and seven medical students gather around the end of the table to observe my doctor performing a pelvic exam, a cervix touch, and a fetal presentation assessment. My pelvis. My cervix. My fetus. The whole scene proceeds impeccably professionally, if it wasn't for the fact that I was not asked to consent to the presence of the students in the room. In this setting, it is simply assumed that the patient agrees to be subjected to student medical practice.[2] Right now, I have no choice but to bear the intruding presence of this cohort of medical students and residents. My vulnerability is simultaneously tamed and amplified by this sudden reification for learning purposes of my pregnant body. That an established and experienced professional takes care of my pregnancy reduces my anxieties. Yet, being examined in a university clinic amounts to being exposed as pedagogic material. The clinical exam ends with the good news that I am not, for the moment, at risk of premature labor. As I leave the hospital, my trust in the care it provides a bit shaken by the lack of concern for my privacy and dignity, I start to wonder about how this consultation would have taken place in "the other hospital."

Here I draw again from my experience of giving birth in a public maternity hospital to show that women navigate competing rationalities when exposed to multiple channels of reproductive care delivery. As I demonstrated in chapter 4, Romanians' relation with state medicine is often fraught with contradictions that are particularly visible in the field of reproductive care. Beside the incomplete reforming of public care, citizens also face the emerging challenges brought about by the privatization of medicine. Exposed to unprecedented choices between public and private reproductive medicine, some women—my impromptu interlocutor and myself included—struggle to produce new definitions of what counts as adequate care and to locate that care in particular institutions. Satisfactory care is often expected from public hospitals, but it is sometimes actively sought for in private ones. Conversely, private clinics may be praised for excellent services, but many would still choose public hospitals despite the substandard care they provide. Women argue against but also fantasize about "the other hospital," the way that Doctor MT and I did. As Romanians learn how to navigate these developing landscapes of reproductive medicine, "the other hospital" switches back and forth between the private and the public one.

In this chapter, I continue to explore the systemic contingencies contributing to Romania's cervical cancer crisis. I consider how women's ideas about adequate sexual and reproductive medicine, including cervical cancer prevention, have been altered by the possibility of accessing forms of care that are not managed by the state. In chapter 4, I showed that, despite the postcommunist transformations of the medical system, women of Delcel still largely consider health a state-defined project. However, women are not oblivious of emergent forms of care beyond state medicine, such as privately owned hospitals or clinics funded by nongovernmental organizations (NGOs). In Romania, as elsewhere, the neoliberal policies pushing for the privatization of medical care drew on visions that linked individual agency to better health outcomes. But this narrative began to lose its hold over both politicians and citizens as problems of quality and affordability of health care were made more apparent. As I demonstrate in this chapter, despite perceiving private maternity hospitals as sites of "stratified reproduction" (Colen 1995) and conspicuous consumption, many women endorsed the alternative of giving birth in a private clinic. Disabused by the shortcomings of care as a social right embodied in state hospitals, they adopted the model of care based on economic privilege, represented by private clinics.

In reality, the boundaries between state and private medicine are quite porous. Patients and doctors alike have developed tactics of steering between public and private care. Referral practices marred by potential conflicts of interests highlight how permeable and unstable are the gray zones between public and private medicine. I feature the story of Călina, who, after giving birth to her first baby in a public maternity hospital in Bucharest, chose a private clinic, also in Bucharest, for her second birth. While Călina's case of shopping around for birthing alternatives is atypical of what women of Delcel actually do, it is not necessarily unusual in terms of what women and their families fantasize about doing. Her story exposes the dynamic of desires and possibilities that govern the quest of reproductive care in contemporary Romania. Building on Călina's case, I also look at the ever-increasing numbers of Romanian women who opt for expensive C-sections in private hospitals. Finally, I return to *Renașterea* mobile clinic to examine the NGO-driven channels of sexual and reproductive care, which exist beyond both state and private medicine. I hypothesize about the unusual silence surrounding the mobile clinic from the otherwise vocal women from Delcel. The NGO-funded clinic may represent to them an ambiguous, unprecedented form of care that muddles the distinctions between private and public medicine and between prevention and cure.

As we shall see, private and NGO-driven alternatives to state medicine expose women to emergent forms of "health citizenship" that include redefining access to care as a consumerist-driven privilege, exerting real agency over reproductive care choices, challenging established patriarchal regimes of health care delivery, and engaging in patterns of mobility that defy rigid, territorial-based distribution of care.

"I URGE YOU TO GIVE BIRTH IN A PRIVATE MATERNITY HOSPITAL"

Paula's doorbell is not working, but there is no need for it because, once I stop in front of her gate, her dog starts barking furiously. All sweaty, her hands covered in mud, Paula shows up from her backyard, hushes the dog, and invites me in, apologizing for losing track of time and forgetting about our interview. It is early April, and Paula has been preparing seedlings for her garden. Slender and tall, she wears black sweatpants and a matching top—a rip-off Adidas training suit, judging by the cheap white nylon strips sewn on the sides of her pants and shirt. She leaves her muddy clogs at the door threshold. I remove my shoes, too. Her house interior, recently renovated, is unexpectedly minimalist, with laminated floors and IKEA furniture. After washing her hands and changing her sweatshirt, Paula pours mineral water for both of us. A plate of cookies—Lent friendly, she assures me—was already waiting for us on the coffee table. Longtime divorced, Paula is fifty years old and lives alone. Her only daughter moved with her husband to Spain a few years ago. Paula works as a store manager for a private local business. If gardening is a subsistence necessity for many of her neighbors from Delcel, for Paula, it is just a hobby or, as she puts it, a "habit."

During our conversation, I ask Paula what advice she would give to an expectant mother. She sits pensively for a moment before telling me: "Well, I don't know. . . . Do you know why I am so in favor of those private clinics?" Surprised by her question, I try to clarify what she means: "Your advice to a future mother would be to go to a private clinic?" Paula then launches into a diatribe: "Yes, yes, there they care; here they don't care. Why on earth care when the doctor has seven million,[3] the same salary as the janitor? Even the subway sweepers have better salaries. Why on earth care?" She continues, mimicking an imaginary doctor addressing an imaginary patient: "I don't have aspirin for you. Here, take the prescription and go buy it. Have you bought it?" My dialogue with Paula took place months before my conversation about "the other hospital" with Doctor MT. In retrospect, Paula's words foreshadowed that later conversation, as she opposed public and private reproductive care by articulating spatial distinctions between *there*, where "they care," and *here*, where "they don't care." As other women, Doctor MT and myself included, Paula perceived the private maternity hospital literally outside her reach, placed in a generic "there," bearing the mark of otherness.

Though vehement, Paula's critique of public maternity hospitals and praise of private ones is not unusual. In the last three decades, the emergence of privately owned OB-GYN care has shaped the Romanian medical landscape and affected public ideas about sexual and reproductive medicine. The first private OB-GYN practices were opened in the early 1990s in urban areas, after the passing of law 31/1990 that authorized the creation of commercial societies, including those aimed at providing medical care. They offered mostly contraception, gyneco-logical exams, and prenatal care. Private OB-GYN clinics, endowed with sophis-ticated surgical theaters and birthing rooms, were developed in the early 2000s, and their number grew significantly after 2007, prompted by the macroeconomic stabilization that followed Romania's joining the European Union (EU). As of 2021, there were over thirty private OB-GYN clinics throughout Romania, offer-ing everything from screenings for sexually transmitted infections (STIs) and cervical cancer prevention to secondary and tertiary gynecological and obstetri-cal care. In Roşiorii de Vede, there was one private OB-GYN practice, run by a doctor who also works as a full-time specialist in the public municipal hospital. Capitalizing on people's perceptions about the low quality of care in state hospi-tals, most private clinics promote their services as better alternatives to public medicine. Paula voiced her uneasiness about state medicine by consistently using "care" (*a păsa*) as a keyword to contrast public and private maternity hos-pitals. Later in the conversation, when I prompted her to consider the scenario of her daughter being pregnant in Romania, Paula resumed her criticism of pub-lic hospitals: "[I would encourage her to go to] a private clinic, for sure. Can't you see? Public hospitals lack everything. No funds, no specialists, very low sala-ries. You get no care there."

When I asked other women from Delcel about the ins and outs of giving birth in private maternity clinics, they noted the presumed superior quality of care that these institutions provided. "People go [to private maternity clinics] because they want to be taken care of, they want to receive attention. If they receive atten-tion, they give birth more easily" (Adriana, age 48). "Private maternity [clinic] has its advantages. I guess they pamper you like a princess during hospitaliza-tion" (Eugenia, age 42). "I don't know anything about private maternity hospi-tals. We have only a public hospital here, but the care might be better in private clinics" (Ioana, age 59). Because I was pregnant with my second child when some of these conversations took place, I was often advised to choose a private clinic for my own delivery: "If your financial situation is good, I urge you to give birth in a private maternity hospital. They care more; they take better care of you and your baby" (Teodora, age 45). "Go there, to the private maternity hospital, and you'll get better care" (Maria, age 74).

While acknowledging the presumably better care that one receives in a private clinic, some women nonetheless emphasized the financial barriers in accessing such forms of privileged medical attention: "They go [to the private maternity hospital] because they have the financial means to get such good care. Of course, I never set foot in there, but I guess the conditions are better" (Ramona, age 49). "I gave birth in a public hospital, but if I had material resources, I would have definitely chosen the private one" (Aurelia, age 35). Remarkably, Ileana (age 59) did not even acknowledge the supposed better care of private clinics, choos-ing instead, in a condescending-sounding comment, to emphasize only social privilege and economic power: "[People go to private maternity clinics] just for the sake of it. Because they have high connections." Care in a private clinic is adequate, yet not granted.

To many Romanians, the cost of care in private maternity clinics is prohibitive. Public maternity hospital deliveries are officially free of charge, regardless of the mother's insurance status. In contrast, as of 2021, a "birth package" (*pachetul de naștere*) in a private maternity hospital—including hospitalization, prenatal and postnatal exams, lab analyses, epidural set or spinal anesthesia, personalized diet, cosmetic products, and lactation counseling—ranged between $1,400 and $2,200, which corresponded to two and, respectively, three average monthly salaries after taxes. A Pap smear was the equivalent of $45, and a human papillomavirus (HPV) test cost about $80.[4] That cervical cancer prevention is offered for a high price tag in private clinics has prompted social scientists to discuss the "commodification of the cervix," first described by Linda McKie in her study among working-class women in 1990s England (1995, 453) and later in relation to Romania's postcommunist medicine (Băban et al. 2005; Todorova et al. 2006). Despite the high costs of care in private maternity clinics, the field of private OB-GYN medicine has been booming. Already in 2010, 10 percent of the babies in Bucharest were born in private maternities (David 2010).

Several younger women, such as twenty-six-year-old Fira, who had no children, contrasted the reliability of the online information about private clinics found on their websites with the volatility of the word-of-mouth usually surrounding recommendations for public hospitals and doctors working in the public system. According to Fira, women giving birth in private clinics were more likely to use the internet to settle on a birthing venue. However, this assertation was not necessarily true in my experience of observing many Delcel residents reading online doctor reviews and online peer advice about navigating care in public hospitals. Other women recommended private maternity clinics to avoid the endemic "corruption" that they believed was taking place in public maternity hospitals. They contrasted the private clinics' transparent fee-for-service system with the hidden informal contributions that are so prevalent in Romanian public hospitals. Anamaria (age 29) summarized this dynamic of payments in an involuntarily rhymed sentence: *Nași cu șpagă la stat /și chitanță la privat* ("[You] give birth with a bribe in state [hospital] and a receipt in private [hospital]"). In recognizing that satisfactory care is provided only in exchange for money, women from Delcel demonstrated their familiarity with reproductive medicine in its lucrative, profit-driven version. As I reveal in chapter 6, the high frequency of informal payments in state reproductive medicine may have accustomed Romanians to the idea that care does not come free of charge—that it has, instead, a price tag. In what appears to be marked continuity rather than opposition between "bribe" and "receipt," the value of reproductive care has become increasingly monetized. That more and more Romanian women locate the value of reproductive care in its financial costs has important consequences to their understanding of free cervical cancer prevention as less valuable, as I suggest later in this chapter.

Yet, women's recognition of the presumed superior quality of care in private clinics was not without reserve. Ramona, Eugenia, and Ioana used grammatical markers of the dubitative mood—which I translated using the idiomatic "I guess" and "might be." Also, Ramona underscored that she had never set foot into a private maternity clinic, and we can read in her words a possible frustration about the barriers to access private care. Similarly, Eugenia's comment about a parturient mother being pampered "like a princess" sounds like a five-star review laced in sarcasm. Even Maria, who at first so openly advised me to seek care in a private maternity hospital, later amended her previous endorsement: "Public [hospital], private [clinic] . . . you know what, Miss Cristina? If a bad thing is meant to happen, then it will happen, no matter where you are." Several other women agreed that the standards of care in a private clinic, although much higher than in a public hospital, did not necessarily grant a better birthing outcome for the mother or the baby: "Well, it is true that accommodation is so much better there [in private maternity hospital], but you are not looking for a five-star hotel; you are looking for a place to give birth safely" (Diana, age 27). Like Doctor MT, Eugenia considered that the doctor's professional reputation was paramount: "The key is the doctor, who is not necessarily better because he works in a private clinic. On the contrary."

As noted above, private medicine has been established only recently in Romania. Until two decades ago, the only institutions where doctors could build a professional reputation were public hospitals. For OB-GYNs and other specialists, a doctor's name was strongly associated with a hospital's established image. Giving up a position in a public maternity hospital in order to work exclusively in a private hospital would entail a loss of symbolic and sometimes even financial capital for many doctors. Switching practice completely to private care would prevent a doctor from capitalizing on the hospital's identity. Also, some doctors acknowledge that state medicine is more professionally challenging, as dealing with diverse pathologies in often underresourced environments of care pushes them to find more creative solutions. That "improvisation" (Livingston 2012) is still a mark of public medicine but not of private care points to the uneven development characteristic of upper-middle-income countries. Although in private clinics salaries are higher, in state hospitals doctors benefit from the informal payments and gratitude gifts they often receive from patients. Further, in the last decade, to fight bribery and to prevent brain drain, the Health Ministry has significantly increased payments for medical staff. Thus, some doctors are reluctant to shift to private medicine completely and permanently (Mihalache 2019). They choose instead to strategically navigate between delivering care in both public and private institutions in ways that, although often amounting to conflicts of interests, are rarely legally recognized in this light. As I show in the next section, the fact that OB-GYNs participate in practices that muddle the distinctions between public and private care further shapes patients' emergent understanding of the new landscapes of sexual and reproductive medicine.

MIX-AND-MATCH CARE

Analysts of postcommunist transformations have pointed out the existence of illicit interdependencies between state and market institutions in health care and beyond. These practices—usually involving the fraudulent reallocation of public resources to the benefit of private businesses—tend to be particularly prevalent in obstetrics and gynecology, where private medicine is often practiced in public settings (Simionescu and Marin 2017). Many OB-GYNs who work in public hospitals also own or work in private clinics. Sometimes, they use public hospitals to recruit patients who they refer for further investigations to their own private practice. Thirty-two women (75 percent of those who shared their reproductive life histories with me) recalled either being referred in person or knowing someone else who had been referred by OB-GYN specialists from the public hospitals of Roşiorii or Bucharest to their own private practices.

Four referral scenarios emerged from my fieldwork observations and interviews. In the first two situations, the family physician refers the patient to a specialist from the public hospital, who either establishes a diagnosis and recommends treatment after giving the patient a full consultation (scenario 1a) or, after a more or less cursory exam, refers the patient to the physician's own private practice or clinic for a thorough consultation (scenario 1b). A third situation is that of the family physician referring the patient to a specialist from a private hospital (scenario 2). Finally, sometimes patients skip the family physician and self-refer directly to a private clinic (scenario 3).

I asked women to assess and compare these scenarios in terms of costs and benefits. Scenario 1a involves no official financial costs, since most public hospitals and clinics have a contract with the National Health Insurance House (NHIH), which covers the cost of medical investigations, provided the patient has contributed to the National Health Insurance Fund. However, especially for patients who commute from rural areas, there are expenses hidden in the cost of transportation to and from the clinic, the out-of-pocket contribution for some of the prescription drugs, and the informal contributions intended for the medical personnel (traditionally in the form of gifts, but more recently undergoing a process of monetization). At its worst, in this referral scenario, after waiting for hours in overcrowded hallways, patients are admitted into decrepit consultation rooms with outdated medical technology or into inadequate hospital accommodation, where they are subjected to consultations by burned-out medical practitioners. At its best, patients benefit from competent examinations by dedicated specialists in newly renovated hospital sections endowed with EU-sponsored medical technology.

In a twist to the sequence described above, in scenario 1b, rather than providing a full consultation, OB-GYN specialists use public maternity hospitals to recruit and refer patients to their private clinics. A first-year medical resident in a public maternity hospital in Bucharest, twenty-five-year-old Camelia talked to me during the Easter break, when she came to visit her family in Roșiorii. Camelia witnessed these public to private referrals on a daily basis. Sometimes, she told me, patients were subjected to extremely long waiting times in crowded hallways and to cursory consultations with worn-out medical equipment. Subsequently, doctors suggested that women return for a consultation to the same specialist but in a very different setting—the private clinic. In most cases, Camelia recognized, doctors were not necessarily ill-intentioned. After all, they had no choice but to use the substandard equipment from public maternity hospitals. A referral to their own private practice may well be in their patients' best interest. Situation 1b includes the costs and benefits of a consultation in a public hospital and adds the costs and benefits of an exam in a private clinic. Unless the private clinic has a contract with the NHIH, the patient must pay the fee-for-service. The fee list is usually on display at the reception area and patients receive a receipt for their payment. In this scenario, patients pay twice: under-the-table during the initial consultation in the public hospital and officially with the fee-for-service in the private one. In some cases, the patients may even contribute three times, if we add the gratitude gift that many give to the family physician when they seek the initial referral. This is why, despite being examined twice, women from Delcel rated this scenario as undesirable. Rather than feeling reassured by the re-referral, they exposed the practice as duplicitous and manipulative. Corina (age 44) confessed: "I find it difficult to trust them [the doctors]. It is odd that they switch their behavior from when they work for the state hospital to [when they work for] the private clinic." From a legal perspective, these practices represent a potential conflict of interest. The Health Ministry has repeatedly and unsuccessfully attempted to limit doctors' duplicitous use of public care resources to the benefit of private practices.

In scenario 2, the family physician can refer a patient directly to a private clinic if that institution has a contract with the NHIH. This happens rarely because the number of private practices and clinics having a contract with NHIH is low.[5] In many ways, this is presumably the ideal referral situation. The benefits of being treated in a private medical facility that has a contract with NHIH are short waiting times, access to recent medical technology, clean and proper consultation rooms, and a thorough examination. Some women emphasized the crucial role of the family doctor in helping them access subsidized private medicine. Vasilica, who is seventy-four years old, had surgery for uterine prolapse in a private hospital in Bucharest. She told me:

Dr. A, our family doctor—have you met her?—she was so nice to me. She told me, "I am going to send you [to a private clinic in Bucharest]; they will take good care of you. You ask your son to make an appointment and to go with you. Don't show up earlier because you will not have to wait. And they have the best ultas-ound [*sic*]."[6] I don't know what I would have done without her! And she didn't accept [my gratitude gift], she made me so upset . . . you cannot find another doctor as good as her!

By referring them to private practices and clinics, the family doctor acts, in some patients' eyes, as a state-affiliated-yet-market-savvy intercessor on behalf of citizens' aspirations to access adequate forms of care. However, not everybody echoed Vasilica's enthusiastic endorsement of that particular family doctor who had enrolled many Delcel residents. Several younger women were more reserved in their appraisal. They alleged that the private clinic manager from Bucharest had offered the family doctor financial incentives in exchange for her state-subsidized referrals. Referrals were to them just a corrupted alliance between family doctors and private practitioners, united in exploiting public resources for their own benefit rather than that of their patients. To make this scenario even less ideal, women mentioned the hidden costs of the informal payments they made to the family physician who—as Irina put it—"was kind enough to send me to a cost-free private [practice]." Vasilica also hinted at offering a gratitude gift to the family doctor who referred her to the private clinic in Bucharest. In light of the other women's allegations, we can only wonder about the reasons behind the family doctor's refusal of the gift.

Finally, scenario 3, in which one self-refers to a private health care facility, includes all the costs and benefits associated with private care. It is also the only scenario that completely skips informal payments, even though, in three out of the four referral scenarios described above, the end point is a private medical care institution.

I asked Camelia about the mechanisms that incentivized doctors to refer their own patients from public to private clinics. She connected the high frequency of practices that muddled the distinctions between public and private medicine to the specific temporality of obstetrical care. Camelia explained that, unlike unplanned emergency care or one-time surgical interventions, obstetric care involved regular prenatal and postnatal exams that spanned over many months. This relatively extended period of care allowed both doctors and patients to be more strategic in the ways they navigated the medical system. In chapter 4, I examined women's engagement with state reproductive medicine as improvised and tactical rather than planned and strategic. However, it appears that private care allows practitioners—and, to a certain degree, women as well—to create strategies within tactics or even to upgrade some tactics to a strategic level. Such was the case of Călina, the only woman among those I interviewed who had given birth in both a state hospital and a private clinic. Her story demonstrates the power of ethnography to pull apart binary oppositions such as that between tactic and strategy and to give us a glimpse into the truly fluid reality of reproductive decision-making.

BIRTHING AROUND

Three years after giving birth to her first son in a Bucharest state maternity hospital, Călina chose a private clinic for her second son's birth. Given her experience with both private and public reproductive medicine, Călina was in a unique position to compare and contrast two different regimes of health care delivery and to provide an informed glimpse into the workings of "the other hospital."

Călina was thirty when she became pregnant with her first child. She found out about Dr. D, a male in his early fifties, from her neighbors, by word-of-mouth. Despite rumors about a malpractice case that was never formally filed as a lawsuit, Dr. D was one of the most celebrated OB-GYN specialists in Bucharest. He was full-time appointed to a public maternity hospital—which was also a teaching hospital—and had a professorship position at the University of Medicine and Pharmacy. In addition to these affiliations, Dr. D owned a private OB-GYN practice. Călina contacted him through an acquaintance who had been his patient. For the first visit, Dr. D instructed Călina to come for a pregnancy test to the ambulatory consultation room of the public hospital. Călina sat in a packed waiting room for about an hour—long enough, she told me, to realize that she may have been the only happily pregnant woman in the crowd. From the conversations she overheard around her, she inferred that all the other women were waiting to get abortions. Călina recalled feeling embarrassed at the thought that she may have been mistakenly taken for someone seeking an abortion as well. Eventually, Dr. D examined Călina and performed a cursory ultrasound examination. Without completing any other clinical examination or laboratory test, he told Călina that everything was fine and gave her his business card, instructing her to make an appointment at his private practice a month later. Călina thanked him and offered him an expensive chocolate box that she had brought with her as a gratitude gift. He accepted the gift, advised her to not carry heavy weights, and then walked her to the door. He bade her goodbye while patting her on the back in a gesture that Călina perceived, in retrospect, as patronizing. During the following months, she commuted from Roșiorii to Bucharest for monthly medical checkups at Dr. D's private practice. Each time she was given an ultrasound exam, and she paid out of pocket the full fee-for-service.

When labor pains kicked in, Călina's father-in-law, a well-connected businessman, immediately called his associates in Bucharest. With their help, he managed to make a reservation for one of the only two "special rooms" for parturient mothers at the public maternity hospital where Dr. D was affiliated. Unlike regular rooms, which were free of charge but had six or seven beds and a bath-room at the end of the hallway, this one had to be paid for but featured only two beds and had its own bathroom. On their way to Bucharest, Călina's father-in-law called Dr. D on his cell phone and told him that she was about to give birth. When they arrived at the hospital, Dr. D was there, although it was past his shift. The birth took place without much pain. As instructed by her doctor, Călina had bought in advance the epidural set and Dr. D administered her the local anesthetic. The moment the baby came out, she heard Dr. D yelling at a nurse, but she was too confused to understand why. Immediately after the baby's birth, the neonatal nurse took the baby to the newborn room, and it would be a couple of hours before Călina was able to see him. She recalled the doctor yelling incident only when she first saw her baby boy and noticed a superficial wound on his forehead. When she asked a nurse about the scratch on her baby's head, she was told that "it was noth-ing." She was kept in the maternity hospital for a couple of days, during which she felt slightly neglected. Dr. D came once a day to check on her, but he was rather distant. Although the hospital practiced rooming-in, nobody showed Călina how to breastfeed. After several failed and painful attempts to feed her baby, Călina asked a nurse for advice, after offering her a five lei bill (about US$1.5). She eventu-ally managed to breastfeed her newborn. However, as she constantly feared that the baby did not get enough milk, once she was released from the hospital, she started to complete his intake with powdered milk. Within a month, the baby was weaned and continued to receive only formula until he turned four months old.

For her second pregnancy, Călina decided to go to Dr. E, a young female OB-GYN who worked in a private maternity clinic in Bucharest. Dr. E was not nearly as famous as Dr. D, but she had a good professional reputation. Călina heard about her from a female coworker. She called the clinic and made an appoint-ment for her first visit. For her initial consultation, she only paid the official fee-for-service. She told me that she felt relief not having to provide a gratitude gift. Dr. E proved to have great communication skills. She explained to Călina everything she was doing and seeing on the ultrasound screen. In contrast to the crowded hallway of the public hospital where she had her first pregnancy checkup, the private clinic's brightly painted waiting room featured ergonomic seats and was equipped with plasma TVs that were strategically loud enough to provide privacy to the patient-doctor conversations. (During my own postpar-tum visit in one private clinic in Cluj, I noticed a setting similar to the one Călina described, with minimalist laminated furniture and health promotion posters featuring stock images of smiling women and babies.)

Aware that the private maternity hospital did not have neonatal intensive care, Călina prepared two different bags a few weeks ahead of her due date. The first bag, made in the hope that the pregnancy would reach the term, contained only her identity card, cell phone, toothbrush, and a debit card. For the second bag, which Călina packed "just in case" of a premature birth in a public maternity hospital, she looked up online checklists for birthing in a state maternity hospital. She packed cotton, diapers, soap, towels, napkins, newborn clothing, powder milk, baby bottle, pacifier, diaper rush cream, tea, toilet paper, a mug, a plate, cutlery, and money in small bills—items similar to the ones in my own hospital bag, which I listed in chapter 4. The birth took place smoothly. The hospital provided the epidural set. Călina paid the final bill in local currency at the registration and received a receipt. The nurses volunteered to help Călina breastfeed and encouraged her to not give up. Călina successfully breastfed her second child until he was twenty-two months old. She never gave him any powdered milk.

While not typical for the women in my study, Călina's story of "birthing around" is nevertheless illustrative of seeking and receiving reproductive health care in contemporary Romania. First, Călina switched from state-subsidized care provided by an authoritative male doctor of established reputation to private and costly care managed by a little-known young female doctor. She made a counterintuitive decision by choosing expensive care over supposedly free care and by accepting to be taken care of by a relatively unexperienced professional instead of an accomplished one. However, as she recalled her birthing experiences, Călina expressed disappointment about her first birth in the public hospital and thorough satisfaction about the second one in the private clinic. When I asked her why she had switched doctors and hospitals, Călina admitted with disarming candor: "For my second birth, I went to the private maternity because I could afford it." However, even for her first birth, Călina and her relatives succeeded to secure better hospital accommodation by mobilizing financial and interpersonal resources. The ability to access higher-quality accommodation did not change much between her two births. It seems that, by consulting Călina in both the public hospital and the private practice, Dr. D exposed her to the limits of public medicine as well as to the possibilities of private care. It is unclear whether Călina's exposure to two different regimes of health care delivery embodied in the same professional affected her subsequent choices. But we know that by the time she switched to a private maternity hospital, Călina had been socialized within the universe of private prenatal care by her state-affiliated doctor.

Second, Călina's contrasting experiences with reproductive medicine are gendered. Her birthing choices become less perplexing when we examine the praise for the communication skills of her younger female doctor and, respectively, the critique of the distant and patronizing attitude of the older male obstetrician. In Romania, private reproductive care tends to embody a less patriarchal and more cosmopolitan alternative to the authoritative and technocratic state medicine. The patriarchy embedded in the provision of sexual and reproductive care was reinforced under communism, when men were trained to become obstetricians in disproportionately higher numbers compared to women. The field of obstetrics and gynecology started to be populated by an increased number of female specialists only in recent decades.[7]

Third, in the light of Călina's experiences, we can distinguish between distinctive practices of materiality that correspond to different regimes of reproductive medicine. The content of the two hospital bags reveals her assumptions about the quality of the care provided in the two settings. The extensive lists of items that she packs for the public birth alternative contrasts with the lightness of the private hospital bag. The symbolic and practical opposition between the use of the bank card for the fee-for-service in the private clinic and the small paper bills for informal contributions in the public hospital are also important. Whereas the card embodies transparent yet impersonal market relations, the paper bills are the means for informal but personalized exchanges. Also, in their descriptions of the private clinic settings, Călina and others anchored historically the material conditions shaping their present experiences in receiving care. The overcrowded hallways and worn-out technology of the public hospital appeared to reproduce past provincial regimes of health care delivery. In contrast, the contemporary design and top-of-the-line technology featured in the private maternity hospital connected Călina as a consumer to a global market of reproductive care services. After all, Călina explicitly emphasized her switching from public to private medicine as consumer-driven rather than anything else. Similar to women's experiences with reproductive medicine in post-Soviet Russia, Călina's "consumer subjectivity" emerges at the intersection between monetary payments for health care and the rethinking of power dynamics between patient and providers (Temkina and Rivkin-Fish 2020). There are other forms of commodification of sexual and reproductive care brought about by the privatization of medicine and by the codependencies between state and private medicine in Romania. One of the most salient is the unprecedented increase in cesarean deliveries on maternal request.

ELECTIVE AND EXPENSIVE: C-SECTION IN A PRIVATE CLINIC

Let us take another glimpse into the workings of "the other hospital," and the ways it has changed women's ideas about the limits and possibilities of reproductive medicine, by briefly examining the increase in elective C-sections—that is, cesarean deliveries "performed at the request of the mother in the absence of any medical or obstetric indications" (Ionescu et al. 2019). According to recent estimates, Romania is the European country with the largest absolute increase in the overall—elective and medical—number of C-sections. From 7.2 percent in 1990, C-section rates increased to 36.3 percent of total births in 2016 (Betrán et al. 2016), with rates as high as 47.2 percent of total births at *Filantropia* Hospital in Bucharest in 2014 and 77 percent of total births at *Spitalul Universitar* in 2017. Some estimate C-sections in private clinics around 60 percent (Simionescu and Marin 2017; Păduraru and Udișteanu 2018).

During the pronatalist decades (1966–1989), doctors were forced to strictly ration surgical deliveries because after two C-sections, women were deemed to be at high risk of not being able to carry to term another pregnancy, and they were granted surgical sterilization (Kligman 1998). Thus, C-sections became sought-after procedures under communism since they allowed women to control their fertility from within the official medical system. Some women attempted, using informal connections and under-the-table contributions, to persuade doctors to falsify their medical records to get approval for a cesarean delivery (Păduraru and Udișteanu 2018). In the light of Romania's recent history of pronatalism, it appears that giving birth via C-section has a lasting association with the ability to secure access to forms of care understood as privileged. Today, state maternity hospitals only grant surgical deliveries based on medical indications and decline women's requests for elective C-sections. In some cases, the old tactics of making informal payments in exchange for a false medical indication are still effective (Tudorică 2017). However, many women would instead choose a private maternity hospital, where they pay the fee-for-service associated with the procedure (Simionescu and Marin 2017).

Although, in theory, elective surgical births are performed at women's request, the reality is that C-section deliveries are often first suggested by obstetricians. In Brazil, the country with of one of the highest rates of C-sections in the world, most of these elective, surgical deliveries are generated by future mothers' desires to preserve their bodies unaltered or their fears of discrimination and poor quality of care, but also by doctors' professional and personal agendas (Hopkins 2000). Similarly, in Romania, doctors may suggest a C-section "guided by the principle that providing a service to their 'client's satisfaction' means keeping 'the client'" (Simionescu and Marin 2017, 9). This is particularly true for surgical births, because a C-section becomes a medical indication for future ones. As Monica (age 29) bluntly explained, "I did not have my daughter through C-section, but I have a lot of friends who did. There are two main reasons: medical complications . . . or the doctor simply recommends this option, as it is the most convenient for him and the patient. It is also the most financially rewarding for doctors."

With malpractice laws finally adopted in 2006, in preparation for Romania joining the EU, OB-GYNs have also become increasingly adept in practicing defensive medicine. Seen by some as a "natural and predictable outcome of free market medicine," defensive medicine reflects "a global intolerance to risk" (Ionescu et al. 2019, 111). A forty-year-old childless family doctor, Aura stated: "I would choose cesarean in a private clinic because I don't need any supplemental worry." Rada, thirty-six years old, who had her baby through a cesarean delivery in a private clinic recalled: "The doctor told me that if I would get a C-section, there would be less surprises. Everything was planned." While Rada seemed to assume that the "surprises" referred to unpredictable outcomes for the birthing mother and her fetus, we can wonder whether her doctor was not also considering his schedule and professional reputation.

In the last decades, some countries have witnessed an increasingly strong move toward natural birthing, sometimes at home or in birthing centers, assisted by doulas and midwives. Such reactions against hospital-managed "technocratic births" (Davis-Floyd 2003) were catalyzed by feminist attempts to reclaim women's power over their own bodies. In Romania, such birthing ideals are at best marginal. Hospital births, including elective C-sections, are overwhelmingly shaping the normative views on giving birth. While feminism is not monolithic, neither as ideology nor in practice, it is nevertheless accurate to state that, in contemporary Romania, most women's tactics in seeking reproductive care are not shaped by feminist agendas. As a possible epitome of choice in reproductive care, elective C-sections align women and doctors to the global values of free market biomedicine. A surgical birth becomes a palpable sign not only of power and status but also of belonging to transnational circuits of consumption. The cesarean section is a way to participate to a connected world, and the private clinic is the place that enables the aspiration to acquire cosmopolitan forms of health citizenship (figure 12).

The experiences and perceptions of reproductive care made possible by the creation of private maternity clinics are relevant to women's responses to cervical cancer prevention. These experiences have shaped women's ideas about postcommunist reproductive medicine in general. Because of their direct or mediated exposure to privately owned maternity care, women from Roşiorii understood contemporary reproductive medicine, in contrast with communist reproductive care, as lucrative and profit-driven, often out of reach to most of them, with access to care conditioned by economic resources. This version of medicine also challenged established patriarchal and local hierarchies and provided women with the opportunity to engage in consumerist practices when accessing health care services. However, in marked continuity with the past regimes of care, present-day reproductive medicine also appears to require astute navigation of muddling boundaries and precarious resources such as neonatal intensive care. The changing landscapes of contemporary reproductive medicine are even more complicated because of additional channels of health care distribution, beyond state and private medical care, represented by NGOs. Let us take a look at how women from Delcel reacted to NGO-provided cervical cancer prevention.

NEVER SEEN BEFORE

In the introduction to this book, I followed the NGO Renaşterea's mobile clinic and its journey from Bucharest to Roşiorii de Vede. I used the clinic's travel to provide readers with a glimpse into the rapidly changing landscapes from an urban cosmopolitan center to a quasi-rural periphery. In my account, I took the

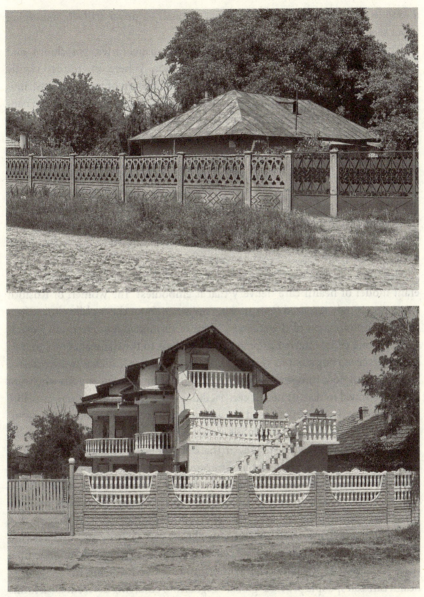

FIGURE 12. Cultural transformation and economic stratification in Delcel. Two neighboring houses on the "Flag-Bearer" street. (Photos by the author.)

readers on a tour of southern Romania to contemplate its people and places from inside the moving mobile clinic. Yet, as the readers and I were watching the shifting scenery, we were also being watched. On the sides of the road, people were staring, quite intently, at this white truck featuring an enormous pink ribbon sticker. To many Romanians, especially the ones living outside the big cities, a mobile clinic is a radical new sighting—literally a novel artifact, something never seen before.[8]

Under communism, access to health care in dispensaries, polyclinics, and hospitals was strictly based on territorial affiliation. Where one resided rigidly dictated the medical facilities one would use. This system of territorial distribution of health care delivery allowed the authorities to exert strict population control that served the ideological goals of pronatalism, among other things. The postcommunist health care reforms have not significantly changed the way policy makers, medical providers, and patients understand the distribution of care. The residents of Delcel had never seen a mobile clinic before the 2010s. Without ice-cream trucks or wandering food vendors in their neighborhood, the only itinerant vehicles that people from Delcel had ever seen were the wagons of the traveling Roma. Marginal and barely tolerated by the authorities, some of the Roma offered tinsmith services, while others sold handmade wooden products, such as barrels, spoons, and coat hangers.

How do Romanians understand the novelty of the mobile clinic and the itinerant model of health care delivery that it embodies? The women of Roşiorii were surprisingly reserved in expressing opinions about the mobile clinic. Even the most opinionated of them stayed silent or dismissed my questions. Worldwide, mobile clinics started as pragmatic solutions to the issue of access to care for underserved populations (Luque and Castaneda 2013). Such was the case, for instance, with poor indigenous Peruvian women from isolated regions who were unable to travel to distant health care facilities. Making a mobile clinic available at the local marketplace increased the women's chances to be screened for cervical cancer (Ferris et al. 2015). Mobile clinics can also expand people's health literacy. Mobile clinics in rural northern Thailand, for instance, increased the number of women getting a Pap test and improved their knowledge about cervical cancer screening (Swaddiwudhipong et al. 1999). It is still unclear whether mobile clinics can produce a more radical mutation in redefining the role of personal agency in accessing health care. However, ethnographic accounts suggest that mobile clinics and, more generally, itinerant health care delivery as a model of care may challenge the normative powers of biomedicine. Occupying "an interstitial space" (Harvey 2011, 51) between traditional and modern medicine, traveling Maya health care salespeople provide "global insights into emerging heterodoxical forms of public health care that contest bio-medical authority and challenge our preexisting definitions of what counts as 'access'" (Harvey 2011, 47).

In contextualizing Delcel residents' silence about the mobile clinic, I suggest that they may have situated the mobile clinic at the intersection between global consumerism, capitalist extraction, and the state's failure to provide adequate medical care. First, people understood that Renaşterea mobile clinic was not a state-affiliated initiative. Since the only alternative to state medicine that they had knowledge of was the care that private clinics provided, they may have collapsed the NGO's mobile clinic and private medicine. As I show in this chapter, for the women of Delcel, the ability to access private reproductive medicine is a form of conspicuous consumption in a global market of health care services. The mobile clinic may have represented to some yet another gateway to global consumerism, with all the benefits and frustrations that women of Delcel associated with such emergent forms of care. That this may have been the case is proved by the reactions to another NGO-coordinated mobile clinic that offered free cervical cancer and breast cancer screenings to a Roma community from northwestern Romania. Part of the reason the Roma women declined preventive care was that they assumed that, since the clinic was not state-affiliated, they would have to pay for the screening it provided, as they would have to pay at a private clinic (Andreassen et al. 2017). Since "medical infrastructures . . . are also defined by intangible, ambiguous, and densely symbolic spectropolitics" (Varley and Varma 2018, 631), the ghost of the private clinic, with its prohibitive fee-for-service, may have similarly haunted the women of Delcel at the sight of the mobile clinic. Even if novel, the mobile clinic was nevertheless evocative of preexistent power relations.

Second, the eventual realization that the medical services of the Renașterea mobile clinic were free of charge may have produced additional perplexities and suspicions. Some women from Delcel may have seen the clinic as a form of capitalist extraction because of its obvious links to transnational values and practices embodied in the very appearance of the shiny white truck with a pink ribbon sticker on its side. By making medical care that is not distributed by the state free of charge, the NGO may have stirred uneasiness about a hidden global market agenda of exploiting local (reproductive) bodies. As I show in chapter 6, many of these women were aware of the tensions between global and local, which they identified mostly in relation to food and foodways. Buying the cheap and allegedly pesticide-laden imported supermarket vegetables was seen by some as surrendering to circuits of global consumption that substituted the reliance on local, more pristine food production. Suspicions about the value of "imported" practices of care could have informed Delcel women's perceptions about the mobile clinic in ways that are perhaps similar to the reactions of Indian parents to the fact that local NGOs were involved in the national HPV vaccination campaign (Towghi 2010, 2013). Because NGOs mediate between global values and local practices, Indian parents refused vaccination in an attempt to protect their daughters' bodies from perceived forms of foreign intrusion to the real benefit of transnational entities.

Finally, people in Roșiorii de Vede may have seen the mobile clinic as evidence that the state had failed them again. In chapter 4, I exposed the extent to which Romanians are struggling to navigate the unstable landscapes of postcommunist state medicine. The presence of the NGO-driven mobile clinic may have only reinforced the conviction that the state is not capable of providing adequate care. The void is occupied by other forms of health care distribution that people may have associated with the market economy. My hypothesis relies on the fact that the women who shared their reproductive stories with me understood intuitively that the "markets stretched the bounds of governmentality" (Ong 2006). They felt abandoned by the state and left at the mercy of the market. Again, the sight of the mobile clinic may have encapsulated more than one evocative apparition, reminding people of their current vulnerability.

The women of Delcel may have perceived the Renaşterea mobile clinic as a gateway to global consumption, a symbol of capitalist extraction, a sign of state failure to care for its citizens, or a combination of any or all of these. Yet, the Renaşterea mobile clinic does not represent any of these, despite its muddled relationship with state authorities (see interlude, part 2). Women's silence about the mobile clinic may reflect their perplexity about imagining a third channel of health care distribution, which is neither the state nor the market. Moreover, their difficulty to situate the NGO's mobile clinic within a specific type of care may be intensified by the lack of integration of medical care in contemporary Romania. State, private, and NGO-affiliated care exist as a patchwork rather than an integrated system. This fact becomes particularly visible when we consider the lack of reliable follow-up care after cervical cancer screening, especially for the most vulnerable and marginal women (Andreassen et al. 2017). According to the Renaşterea Foundation website, since 2009, more than 16,000 low-income women have received free cervical cancer screenings in the form of Pap smears and free mammograms in the Renaşterea mobile clinic.[9] While these numbers are notable for an NGO project, the mobile clinic's reach has been quite limited. Also, it is unknown how many of these women accessed any form of follow-up care after being diagnosed with an abnormal smear.

HEALTH CITIZENSHIP

I hypothesize that the women from Delcel may have perceived the mobile clinic as the embodiment of an ambiguous model of health care delivery. Their difficulty in vocalizing opinions about the clinic may also reflect the rapid transformations of the ways they understand their "health citizenship" status. Originating in the aftermath of the French Revolution, "health citizenship" is a category of belonging that has been shaped, over time, by the dialectics between health care entitlements and responsibilities, as highlighted through various regimes of governance and welfare (Porter 2011). A particular case of health citizenship is "biological citizenship," a term coined by Adriana Petryna (2003) in her study about Ukrainians navigating post-Chernobyl health care entitlements. While the latter designates asserting personhood by claiming benefits based on the appropriation of suffering, health citizenship entails a consumption and decision-making behavior stemming from awareness of the personal rights to health care.

In postcommunist Romania, health citizenship has emerged, at least in intention, as a market-shaped category of belonging as the country transitioned from socialized to insurance medicine (Bara et al. 2002). The neoliberal assumptions (Harvey 2007) that have guided the privatization and reforming of medical care recast patients as savvy consumers of health care services and dynamic participants in a new culture of health care rights, claims, and belonging. Once in a position to choose among multiple health care options, people are assumed to make rational, optimal decisions for their health that would promote the workings of the liberalized medical system. Individuals and health care institutions would coexist in a mutually profitable relationship. In Romania's new political context, health citizenship would amount to people's deliberate and knowledgeable participation to a liberalized market of health care services, as illustrated by Călina's "birthing around" or by the increase in elective C-sections in private clinics.

The neoliberal ethos intended to redefine health citizenship produced complicated landscapes when medical care was reformed. In August 2011, a presidential law proposal aimed at privatizing the majority of public hospitals. The project triggered heated public debates about the very nature of health care and exposed the inherent contradictions of liberalized medicine (Chirculescu 2011; Domnişoru 2011; Paveliu 2011; Stillo 2011; Raţ 2011). Analysts claimed that "like education, health care cannot be privatized" because it is "too important to be left at the mercy of the market" (la cheremul pieţei) (Paveliu 2011). Some conceded to the privatization of some medical subfields (Vlaston 2011) but argued in favor of state control over laboratory, radiology, and obstetrics (Paveliu 2011; Raţ 2011) and forcefully rejected the privatization of TB sanatoriums (Stillo 2010, 2011; Chirculescu 2011).

The fields of medicine considered unsuitable for privatization are, therefore, TB treatment, medical imaging, laboratory medicine, and reproductive medicine. What these specialties seem to have in common is that the state has a vested interest in maintaining control in various forms. With multidrug-resistant TB endemic to Romania and neighboring countries, state-owned sanatoriums could help confine contagion through centralized care. With radiology and laboratory medicine as adjacent to virtually all other fields of medicine, state would presumably have a lucrative interest.

Those who oppose the privatization of reproductive care hold the postcommunist state responsible for protecting the next generation of Romanians. The concern over privatization is more ideological than practical, with the state still understood as a reliable source of welfare and free care. These concerns produced additional controversies, as some analysts saw the state's monopoly over obstetrics as a continuation of the communist practices of monitoring women's (pregnant) bodies. As I demonstrated in chapter 4, when it comes to assessing the postcommunist state's role in protecting their health and well-being, many

Romanians feel stuck between "too much" and "not enough." In intention, health citizenship in its postcommunist version entails taking calculated decisions aiming for the best health outcomes. In reality, "the development of a consumer subjectivity without a concomitant political subjectivity" (Temkina and Rivkin-Fish 2020, 342) has left health citizenship suspended somewhere between bold claims and meager benefits and between confusing choices and unfulfilled expectations.

CONCLUSIONS

In addition to the postcommunist reforming of state medicine, the privatization of health care brought about a multiplication of the channels through which medical care is delivered. In this chapter, I have shown that being exposed to forms of care beyond state medicine—such as privately owned or NGO-driven clinics—has shaped women's ideas about sexual and reproductive care. From their direct or mediated interactions with private reproductive care, women understood that, as emerging global citizens, patients can increasingly act as consumers and shop around for elective medical interventions, and that male doctors no longer have the monopoly over OB-GYN care. Women also learned that the value of adequate care resides mostly in its often-prohibitive price tag, and that, rather than protecting their well-being, the state would engage in murky forms of complicity with private providers to the benefit of the latter. The lessons that women internalized through their exposure to forms of care beyond state reproductive medicine have produced, in some cases, empowering attitudes about access to care and, in some other instances, frustrations and perplexities about the unsettling landscapes of postcommunist medicine. Already forced by the changing historical circumstances that led to reforms and privatization to reassess the value of sexual and reproductive care, women chose to ignore free cervical cancer prevention when it came right to their door by way of the novel NGO-managed mobile clinic. As one of Kristen Ghodsee's Bulgarian friends said, reflecting on the fast pace of postcommunist transformations in eastern Europe: "enough change for one lifetime" (2011,153).

6 · LOCATING CORRUPTION

This is one of the most dreadful tragedies in the entire history of the Romanian medical system.*

Tufts of brown hair stuck to his sweaty forehead, visibly uncomfortable in his tied-up summer suit, Minister of Health Cseke Attila holds a press conference. As he utters this unnerving statement in front of a table covered with a dozen microphones, the gloomy-looking undersecretary Raed Arafat, who sits next to Cseke, avoids eye contact with the journalists. The previous day, August 16, 2010, the neonatal intensive care unit (NICU) of Giuleşti Maternity Hospital in Bucharest was left unattended by medical staff for approximately forty minutes. During that time, a short circuit in the air-conditioning installation started a fire that destroyed the ward. Eleven premature newborns were severely burned and six of them eventually died (Dobreanu, Gherguţ, and Pocotilă 2010). As they answer the journalists' frenzied questions, both Cseke and Arafat are aware that what makes Giuleşti case especially catastrophic is that less than a year earlier, a similar tragedy had occurred. In November 2009, a nurse from the neonatal section of Bucur Maternity Hospital in Bucharest had placed a healthy newborn girl who had physiological jaundice into an incubator and then forgot about her. The newborn, who was exposed to phototherapy for far longer than she should have, suffered very serious burns. She survived but required several plastic surgeries (Grigore 2009).

Tragic as it was, the incident at Giuleşti Maternity Hospital came as no surprise to the women from Delcel. Many of them recognized in both the Bucur and Giuleşti cases instances of state medicine failing to provide reasonable care to ordinary people. However, most women were not concerned as much with the precarious medical endowment of public hospitals and the risks that medicine practiced in inadequate conditions would pose to the health and well-being of women, expectant mothers, and newborns. As they made an inventory of the facts and rumors surrounding the Bucur and Giuleşti cases, Delcel residents considered details such as the nurses experiencing burnout from frequent thirty-six hour shifts, the fire starting as a consequence of laxly enforced safety rules, the faulty wiring installed by an impromptu electrician, and the astonishingly long absence from the NICU of any medical worker. A "defining feature of bio-medicine" in developing countries, improvisation requires a pragmatic adjusting of established knowledge and practice to the actual means of health care delivery (Livingston 2012). But to the women from Roşiorii, improvisation was deeply immoral. They looked at the Bucur and Giuleşti incidents through a moral lens and highlighted how neglect, poor management, and lack of accountability shaped the provision of health care in public hospitals. The keyword that emerged repeatedly from their comments was corruption (*corupţie*). To them, the ultimate cause of the accidents was the endemic moral corruption surrounding the quest for and the delivery of health care in Romania.[1]

Corruption narratives tend to infuse private and public discourses, especially in contexts of unsettling political, economic, and cultural transformations worldwide. (For India's experience, see Gupta [1995] and Gupta and Sharma [2006]. For Nigeria, see Smith [2008], and for Niger and Senegal, see Blundo and Olivier de Sardan [2006]. For Cuba, see Andaya [2009], and for Russia, see Ledeneva [2006] and Rivkin-Fish [2005].) Gupta recalls that "doing fieldwork in a small village in North India . . . [he] was struck by how frequently the theme of corruption cropped up in the everyday conversations of villagers" (1995, 375). His account would adequately reflect my own fieldwork experience if I replaced "North India" with "southern Romania." Since 1989, the country has experienced political, economic, and cultural change that brought about new entitlements but also burdens and unfulfilled aspirations for ordinary citizens. To Delcel residents, some of these contradictions were particularly visible in the realm of reproductive medicine and its moralities. Women expressed their anxieties about the emergent regime of reproductive health care delivery by identifying corruption as its distinctive feature. To Maria, Ileana, Sorana, Ana, and many other women from Roşiorii, the public maternity hospital epitomized the corrupt condition of the entire medical system and of society at large. As microcosms of the wider society, hospitals provide a glimpse into the way power works to produce knowledgeable experts and docile patients (Foucault [1963] 1994). Women's comments about corrupted care in maternity hospitals were part of broader reflections about the society's workings, revealing once again that "to a great extent, talk about the body and about sexuality tends to be talk about the nature of society" (Scheper-Hughes and Lock 1987, 20). While corruption narratives can encapsulate everyday "naturalized" rapports, for the women in Delcel, corruption became a category to critically think about emerging postcommunist realities. Corruption provided them with an "arena through which the state, citizens, and other organizations and aggregations come to be imagined" (Gupta 1995, 376).

In this chapter, I follow women's concerns with the moralities—rather than the medical circumstances—of reproductive health care. These intense moral anxieties over reproductive medicine are part of the systemic contingencies that have produced the cervical cancer crisis. By delegitimizing medicine on moral grounds,

women hinder cervical cancer prevention from becoming authoritative knowledge. I highlight the ways in which corruption becomes, in lay discourses about
reproductive health as well as in everyday practices of accessing reproductive care,
an all-encompassing designator for state reproductive medicine. The women of
Delcel articulate the relationship between reproduction and corruption through a
multiplicity of narratives about governance and medical care delivery. They would
often integrate rumors and cherry-pick information from mass media into their
personal experiences with reproductive medicine. I aim to disentangle the three
main sources of these narratives about corruption and reproduction in sections
about mass media accounts of reproductive care, people's experiences with reproductive medicine, and rumors of corruption loosely surrounding reproduction.

First, I consider mass media discourses about corruption-ridden reproductive care. I am interested in the potential of media accounts about reproductive
medicine to induce and reinforce women's sense of reproductive vulnerability.
Building on the Romanian language's already profuse idioms of corruption, the
mass media provide citizens with the language to express anxieties over emerging medical landscapes. Second, in recalling a subjective experience of corruption as a tactic to secure privileged access to reproductive care, I include an
account of my own exposure to reproductive medicine as an expectant mother
contingently forced to seek urgent care. I then feature some of the informal practices that people use when navigating state reproductive medicine. Often seen as
normative, these practices are crucial in defining the moralities of reproductive
care for both patients and medical workers. Third, gossip and rumor also shape
people's ideas about corruption and reproduction. I review some of the rumors
that locate corruption and reproduction in relation to food discourses and environmental anxieties. Spread as urban legends, these rumors often originate in
selective readings of mass media accounts. Finally, I look at the particular demographic group of the parents and grandparents of the prepubescent girls who
were targeted for the human papillomavirus (HPV) vaccination. I show how
parental anxieties about their daughters' virginal bodies are informed by a mix of
media discourses about corrupted reproductive care, by rumors about corruption and reproductive bodies, and by the immediate experience of corruption
within the realm of reproductive medicine. I argue that cervical cancer prevention programs such as HPV vaccination provided Romanians with the opportunity to use the idiom of corruption to locate ubiquitous (Gupta 1995) yet volatile
ideas about reproduction and to express their conflicting views on postcommunist reproductive medicine.

. . . AS SEEN ON TV

Both the Giuleşti and Bucur accidents received extensive media coverage and
triggered heated debates about the dismal condition of state medicine and

public reproductive care. In TV shows, newspaper articles, op-eds, essays, and blog posts, experts and nonexperts alike glossed over the tragic events, highlighting the failure of state reproductive medicine to care for the most vulnerable citizens—the newborn (Mixich 2010; Dobrescu 2010; Dobreanu, Ghergut, and Pocotilă 2010; see also Andrei, Efrim, and Gheorghiță 2011; Ionescu 2015). Some reviewed the worn-out material infrastructure of state hospitals, while many others highlighted the moral failures of reproductive medicine. One of the most emotional reactions to the Giuleşti incident came from Mircea Cărtărescu, a celebrated writer and occasional political analyst. Cărtărescu published an article titled "The Massacre of the Innocents" (*Uciderea pruncilor*) in reference to the biblical episode of mass infanticide by Herod the Great. Drawing from his own experience of having had his children born at Giuleşti hospital, the writer saw the accident as the inevitable consequence of shortages, corruption, and neglect.

> The tragedy that has just happened at Giuleşti . . . was destined to happen one day. Giuleşti maternity hospital has been a place of horror, desolation, and material scarcity for the last twenty-three years, when I first stepped inside it. Instead of improving, things got worse there. I cannot forget the dirty rooms lacking hot water, the painkiller shortages, the new mothers having to walk all the way down the stairs to see their husbands just hours after giving birth, the nurses and midwives with their pockets full of wrinkled bills, the doctors scolding women in labor so loudly that you could hear them from the hallways: *Why are you screaming? You liked it when you banged; you should like it now!* I cannot forget the newborns in incubators, the Band-Aids brutally pulled off from their eyelids. For my wife, giving birth at Giuleşti has remained the most shocking and bitter experience of her entire life.

Cărtărescu went on to contrast the poor care provided in Giuleşti Maternity Hospital to a mother's unconditional nurturance, which, he claimed, was universal. He then concluded that Romanians were disdainful barbarians, incapable of protecting future life (Cărtărescu 2010).

In a context of declining fertility rates (Brădăţan and Firebaugh 2007), Cărtărescu's article, as well as the subsequent tabloidization of the Bucur and Giuleşti cases, escalated public anxieties about reproductive vulnerability and corrupted medicine. Postcommunist mass media have routinely reported on fictive hospitalizations and theft from hospitals, pharmacies, and dispensaries and on doctors conditioning care to receiving under-the-table payments.[2] Such accounts have informed people's expectations of receiving adequate care as conditioned by the ability to make informal contributions, within and beyond the field of reproductive medicine. Since 1989, infant and maternal mortality rates have significantly decreased in Romania. At the time of the Giuleşti incident in 2010, in only one decade the country's infant mortality rate had halved, plummeting from 18.6 to 9.8 deaths for 1,000 live newborns. While statistics showed that it had never been safer to give birth in Romania, the women from Delcel saw state maternity hospitals the way Cărtărescu described them, as "place[s] of horror, desolation, and material scarcity." The terrifying image of a maternity hospital nestling death instead of nurturing life was evidence enough to them of the wretched condition of reproductive medicine.

As reflected by mass media, reproductive care was marred by corruption, and taming reproductive vulnerability required one's savvy participation in these very circuits of corruption. When I asked her about the appropriate informal contribution to the medical staff for a public hospital birth, Maria, who, years after the monetary reform still used the old currency in her estimate, evaluated it to be "as much as you can offer, about ten million." I raised my eyebrows in silent perplexity because the amount she mentioned was close to $300. She further elaborated: "Yes, this is the price for a C-section, but you have to bargain, you know? You bargain with the doctor. Things are not as they used to be. Everything is upside down. They show on TV poor, desperate women looking for medical care." One of Maria's neighbors, Gabriela, also linked informal payments to a sense of reproductive vulnerability that she developed from watching the news. Gabriela followed up on her statement from chapter 4—namely, that "all you hear on TV is that mothers die in childbirth, in a hospital, with doctors, with specialists"—with the remark that "you have to give [an informal contribution]." Both Maria and Gabriela backed up their knowledge about informal payments for reproductive care with media accounts of reproductive vulnerability. For them, mass media connected the dots between reproductive vulnerability and corruption. Attempting to denounce corruption and to purify the public sphere, mass media inadvertently promoted it. The medicalization of reproduction had already removed intimate reproductive events from domestic private spaces. With an audience-craving media, hospital births gone wrong have the power to shape the perceived reproductive vulnerability of broader, unrelated audiences. Maria and other women from Delcel extended to cervical cancer prevention the sense of reproductive vulnerability and the mistrust in state medicine that they learned on TV. Several women who recalled having first heard about the HPV vaccine on national TV also claimed those initial media reports were about the vaccine's alleged failures.

IDIOMS OF BRIBERY

The Romanian language has a remarkable lexical diversity for designating informal contributions and connections. *Peșcheș* or *bacșiș*, derived from Arabic via Turkey and originating during the Ottoman rule, refer to a gift or a sum of money that high officials would give in order to secure the sultan's protection. The terms are used today to designate an unofficial gift, in nature or money, offered to an influential person in exchange for personal benefits (DEX 1998). *Bacșiș* means a "tip" as well. *Plocon*, derived from Slavonic, has a similar meaning—a gift made to elicit a personal favor from a powerful individual (DEX 1998). Also a Slavonic word, *mită* is the generic term for bribe, while *şpagă*, derived from the Serbian špag ("pocket"), is the most informal register to refer to a bribe (Zafiu 2010).

Relying on personal connections and informal payments to secure privilege has continued long after the end of the Ottoman rule in 1878. Under the communist economy of "organized shortages" (Verdery 1996), informal practices reemerged with such frequency that new words were created to map them out more thoroughly. One such term is *pilă*, literally meaning "file" (as in "the tool used to file") and employed to designate an influential person. The plural *pile* refers to illicit support given by influent person(s) (DEX 1998). There are two idioms about *pilă/ pile*: one either struggles to get the protection of an influential person (*a avea pile*) or one abusively intercedes in somebody's else favor (*a pune/a băga o pilă*). The use of *pile* under communism was so widespread that one of the most subversive jokes of the 1980s was to read the acronym of the Romanian Communist Party (PCR) as standing for "*Pile—Cunoştinţe—Relaţii*" (influential persons—connections—links/networks). While circumventing official channels was "central to the Socialist system's very functioning" (Rivkin-Fish 2005, 211), informal contributions and connections continued to play a crucial role in people's strategies of accessing health care after 1989. Despite economic and political changes, in post-Soviet Cuba (Andaya 2009) and post-Soviet Russia (Rivkin-Fish 2005), the "ideology of the gift" has persisted along with the transparent payments promoted by emergent market economies. The endurance of informal payments in postcommunist (and postcolonial) contexts amounts to a cultural failure of neoliberalism because it challenges teleological assumptions about liberalized markets and their radically new moralities (Blundo and Olivier de Sardan 2006). Whether informal payments in the field of medical care are pervasive despite or because of reforms (Friedman 2009), they reveal that patients and medical staff are still bound by the tacit rules of a moral economy, even if encapsulated within a market economy.

To the women from Roşiorii de Vede, the idioms of bribery, gifts, and informal connections are essential cognitive and practical tools in their quest for health care. They see the medical encounter between doctor and patient as a locus of uncertainty, marked by an "asymmetric structure of power relations" (Zerilli 2005, 96). To earn the attention of the medical staff, patients deploy tactics that enhance their visibility: "I give the doctor the envelope, and he pays more attention to me" (Ioana, age 59); "Before the consultation, I look into my purse [for the gift or money] and wait to see if he pays attention to me" (Teodora, age 45). Ileana also highlights the imperative of giving: "You cannot go to the doctor empty-handed. If you do so, you don't feel comfortable and he will not pay too much attention to you. You have to make a payment of some kind."

Don't even think not to! Some attention, a bag of coffee, a box of chocolate, flowers. At least slip something into his pocket" (Ileana, age 59).

Seventy-four-year-old retired farmer Vasilica admits: "People offer money. If
you don't offer money, the doctor will not even notice you." She then points to
my notebook: "Write it down. If you don't contribute, he will not notice you!"
Vasilica reflects for a few seconds before adding: "You also have to offer a present
with flowers." Paula, now fifty years old, recalls the informal contributions she
made for her delivery: "I had to give for my planned C-section, so I was prepared, although I had been this OB-GYN's patient for seven years. But this is the
custom. [If you give] you have an additional guarantee [of good care]."

Patients' struggle for visibility is acknowledged by health care providers. Camelia, a young medical resident, pondered about people offering unofficial gifts and
payments: "They want to be sure we pay attention to them. They feel they should
stand out." Attention shapes the medical encounter for both patients and medical workers. Patients aim to receive (be given) attention, while providers will or
will not pay (give) attention to their patients. Originally a rather abstract concept, *attention* has become another central term of reference to informal contributions. In a medical care context, attention is an actual entity that is part of a
reciprocal exchange. The word is even used, as a countable noun to designate a
material occurrence of an informal payment/gift. Adriana (age 48) summarizes
what she perceives as the immutable mechanisms of informal contributions for
health care: "This is the custom. You give [the doctor] something, an attention
[*o atenție*], the envelope. It has been like this since forever. This is the way things
work."

As I was about to learn for myself, the purpose of "the attention" in the form
of an under-the-table contribution is to elicit the doctor's attention to the fact
that the patient needs attention.

. . . AS EXPERIENCED FIRSTHAND

September 2006, Delcel, Roșiorii de Vede. Four months into my pregnancy, I
wake up with a sharp abdominal pain. Panicked and confused, I ask my host,
Ileana, about getting a specialized medical exam. The local dispensary, I am told,
was closed five years ago, after the general practitioner had retired and no one
replaced him. But the municipal hospital has an OB-GYN doctor, and in case of
serious trouble, Bucharest is only a two-hour drive away.

Once I decide to go and see the OB-GYN at the hospital, a whole network of
connections is set in motion. Ileana calls an acquaintance who knows one of the
nurses from obstetrics. Through this channel, the nurse is informed about my
intention to seek an immediate checkup. Luckily, she is on shift this morning, so

I am instructed to rush to the hospital where she will introduce me to the doctor. Before leaving, Ileana hands me two packs of cheap cigarettes, one fancy chocolate box, and two small bags of ground coffee—all intended as gifts for the medical workers and others in exchange for privileged attention. I slip them in my bag, suddenly perplexed to realize the power that informal practices bestow on such ordinary items.

Because my host family does not have a car, one of the neighbors was summoned to drive me to the hospital. When he drops me off, I offer him a pack of cigarettes and the small coffee bag to thank him for the service rendered. He takes the cigarettes but refuses the coffee, telling me that I might need it later. As a novice in the art of reciprocal exchanges, I have just overdone it, but he doesn't capitalize on my faux pas—most likely, I imagine, to not ruin his rapport with Ileana. I step out from the car and stare at the ugly four-story concrete building in front of me. The hospital yard is the very image of desolation and abandonment. The lawn hasn't been mowed in a long time, and scattered empty plastic bottles lie here and there in the weeds. As I find my way to the main entrance, a pack of five or six dogs come barking at me. I am scared, but then I remember an old trick from childhood in the countryside. I stoop down, pretending to pick up a pebble. I mimic throwing the imaginary pebble toward the dogs. They stop short but continue to bark. I am still frightened. The hospital doorman comes out of his cabin and hushes the dogs. I tell him, as instructed by Ileana, that I am expected by Nurse K from the OB-GYN section. The doorman lets me in before I get to hand him any of the gifts I carry in my bag.

The elevator is not working. As I reach by foot the third level, I notice a janitor swiftly mopping the floor. The hallway smells strongly of disinfectant. A few women are waiting, standing in the darkness of a windowless hallway. I find Nurse K in the OB-GYN emergency room. She glances at me, bored, but after I introduce myself and mention Ileana's acquaintance, she immediately becomes friendly. She asks about my gestational age and symptoms but tells me that Doctor N cannot see me right now. A sanitary inspection is expected and everybody is stuck in cleaning activities. While I wait in the hallway, I overhear the janitor telling one of the patients that this was meant to be a snap, surprise inspection, but the inspectors themselves called to warn hospital officials about their imminent visit. Their notice has provided enough time for staff to clean up the OB-GYN section so that it will meet the sanitation standards recommended by the European Union.[3]

After waiting for almost an hour, Nurse K ushers me into Doctor N's consultation room. She tells me that I am "lucky" (*norocoasă*) to be the first patient to be checked immediately following the sanitary inspection. All the medical instruments have just been disinfected, the gynecological table has brand-new cover sheets, and the floor has been thoroughly cleaned. She whispers into my ear: "Be nice to Mr. Doctor!" (*Fii drăguță cu dom' doctor*) before introducing me to Doctor N. He is a short, slim, gray-haired man about fifty-five years old. After asking me a few questions about my pregnancy, he performs a pelvic examination and then an ultrasound check, without uttering, during all this time, any other word. The ultrasound machine is worn-out. It has only a small screen for the doctor's use, which is placed at such an angle that I cannot see anything. Doctor N gazes silently at the screen for five long minutes, during which time my mind runs one catastrophic scenario after another. I interpret his silence as a bad sign. I try to stay calm and silent in order not to ruin his frowned focus. Finally, he turns to me. The pain, he ventures, is probably muscular cramps, for which he prescribes me a supplement of magnesium and vitamin B6. He then offers to reveal the sex of the fetus. I decline, because his long silent stare at the screen has made me doubt his expertise. I tell him that I would leave the pleasure of unveiling this information to my regular OB-GYN. I leave the room without finding the right moment to offer him the chocolate box. Nurse K is waiting for me in the hallway. I tell her that I failed to give the doctor the gift. She offers to do it on my behalf. I hand her the chocolate box and the coffee bag, asking her to forward to the doctor the most appropriate item and to keep for herself the other gift.

Upon returning to Ileana's place, I jotted down field notes. The whole experience left me ashamed, uneasy, and frustrated. As someone studying the changing landscapes of postcommunist reproductive medicine, I was ashamed to realize the extent to which I had taken for granted the care I could access in my native city of Cluj, in northern Romania. Up to that moment, most of my previous experiences with reproductive medicine had taken place in an urban area with a mix of public and private providers. I was used to openly communicating with a doctor who was expertly handling state-of-the-art ultrasound technology. By contrast, Doctor N's taciturn and clumsy use of the worn-out ultrasound machine made me mistrust his expertise. Yet, Doctor N had started the consultation with a pelvic exam, a step that my technologically skilled doctor from Cluj systematically skipped.

The unwelcoming pack of dogs and the unkempt condition of the hospital building made me uneasy. I was tempted to read these infrastructural realities as metaphors for the state of public medicine in Romania (figure 13). However, during conversations with Roșiorii de Vede residents, I came to realize that, to many of them, stray dogs, overgrown lawns, and chipped walls were familiar embodiments of historical continuities between the communist and the postcommunist era. The shiny OB-GYN private clinic I was attending in Cluj would have been as intimidating and foreign to them as the Roșiorii de Vede Municipal Hospital was to me. The cleaning of the section in anticipation of the sanitary inspection provided a particularly interesting perspective on the historical connections between past, present, and future. The ideological intention behind the cleaning was to align the local hospital to transnational standards of hygiene, enforced as a requirement for Romania's imminent joining of the European

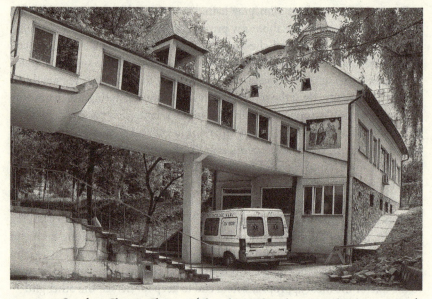

FIGURE 13. Oncology Clinic in Cluj, 2021. (Photo by Pavel Bardă, reprinted with permission.)

Union. For the brief moment surrounding the inspection, one could sense the emergent specter of a clean western European hospital. However, the immediate purpose of the sanitation procedures was purely practical—avoiding a fine for noncompliance. Improving the actual quality of health care delivery was an incidental by-product of the hasty cleaning, not its main purpose, as intended. That the cleaning of the section happened just because of the sanitary inspection pointed to another ghost, this one from the past—the persistence of informal connections and the role they played in hospital management.

The personal connections and the gift giving secured me a timely consultation. From Delcel residents' stories, I was familiar with the centrality of informal practices in the quest for health care, especially with the trope of the nurse acting as an intercessor between patients and doctors. However, I felt frustration over my obvious lack of experience with such practices. Overall, my sense of agency shifted back and forth between powerful and powerless. My worries about my bodily symptoms were overshadowed by my anxieties of properly navigating these networks of balanced reciprocity with everybody from the driver and the doorman to the nurse and the doctor.

. . . AS EVERYDAY PRACTICE THAT MITIGATES REPRODUCTIVE VULNERABILITY

Ileana has invited Ana and her sister-in-law, thirty-five-year-old Crina, to her place. It's a rainy September afternoon and we all sit around a coffee table covered with a plastic cloth, in Ileana's "front house"—the room reserved for guests. We left our shoes on the threshold, and our bare feet are uncomfortable on the itchy nylon carpet. Ileana brings Turkish coffee and store-brought cookies. We talk about informal contributions for medical care. Ana claims that, regardless of the official co-payment, it is customary "to offer something" to the doctor. She enumerates: "A coffee bag, a chocolate box. I usually give coffee. I also give coffee to my kids' teacher at school." Crina adds, in an innocent voice: "I like to give flowers." Ana replies immediately, with a smirk: "It is called bribe [*mită*]." Given my missteps in placing the gifts during my recent pregnancy checkup at Roşiorii de Vede hospital, I ask Ana and Crina about the right time to offer contributions. Crina firmly believes that the offering should happen before the consultation, but Ana favors a more flexible approach: "When you feel it's the best moment." Ana then justifies the use of what she has just labeled bribery: "This is the custom. If you don't contribute, nobody will give a damn—not even the devil [*nu se uită nici dracu' la tine*]." Laughing, she points to the notebook on my lap: "Don't forget to write devil with capital D!"

To Ana and Crina, the gifts offered to medical staff were crucial in ensuring visibility and securing adequate health care. Giving, they felt, was a common social practice that they could not denaturalize, even if they were aware of the illicit character of informal contributions. Ana and Crina did not feel conflicted. They simply recognized informal contributions as means to an end, woven in the texture of customary social interactions. Informal payments in exchange for privileged medical attention remain common both within and beyond sexual and reproductive medicine (Balabanova and McKee 2002, 243; Bara et al. 2002; Al-Khatib, Robertson, and Lascu 2004; Fărcăşanu 2010).[4]

While informal contributions are prevalent in virtually all fields of medicine in contemporary Romania, in reproductive care they have traceable historical roots in a moral economy of gift offerings to traditional midwives (Zerilli 2005). Several women from Delcel still recalled the "old customs" surrounding birth. As previously noted, Adriana became a grandmother when her twenty-seven-year-old daughter gave birth to a son. Adriana compares her own postpartum experience, managed by her own mother, to her daughter's. Her account provides a glimpse into the historical transformations of gift exchanges surrounding birth that span over three generations: "[When I gave birth] my mom baked bread and brought it to the midwife, after birth, with a towel and a small soap. She brought bread, 'cause it brings good luck to the child, and a small soap and a towel for the midwife, to clean herself after helping with the birth. When you give birth, you bake bread for the midwife. This is the custom from the old times, from the countryside."

However, the custom of offering homemade bread, soap, and a towel has waned in recent years. Adriana recalls the recent birth of her grandson: "When my daughter gave birth, we didn't give any bread. My parents did, when I gave birth twenty-seven years ago. Not nowadays, though. For my grandson, we gave [the midwife] a bag of coffee beans and we thanked her. We also gave her 100,000 lei [$3]. Today is not like it used to be; there are no more old customs."

The ceremonial gift giving to the midwife derived from ancient votive offerings (Gal and McKee 2005). The dough rising and the bread baking are metonyms for the baby's growing in the womb. Although they had some economic value, the towel and the soap were foremost symbols of purity and cleanliness. After the medicalization of births in the 1950s, the hospital midwife—or the anesthesiologist, in case of C-section—was still offered these traditional items, along with other gifts.

Adriana's account points to more than the transition from ritual offerings of homemade bread to store-bought commodity items. In addition to the coffee bag, she offered a small amount of money to the midwife who helped with her grandson's birth. In Romania, as elsewhere in postcommunist contexts, informal contributions have undergone increased monetization (Rivkin-Fish 2005). The invisibility of the money (often enclosed in an envelope) grants the patient visibility (Praspaliauskiene 2016). The monetization of bribery demonstrates that, in parallel with resisting change, corruption also accommodates the transformations brought about by the free market consumerist practices that are dependent on cash flows (Ledeneva 2006). While the transparent fee-for-service is paid in local currency, informal payments are often made in foreign currency, most commonly in euros, reflecting precisely this transnational consumerist ethos. Whether under the form of gifts or money, informal contributions remain quasi-invisible. In their descriptions of the bodily techniques they used when placing under-the-table contributions, women emphasized how they would either discreetly slip the envelope into a medical worker's pocket or unobtrusively hand the bagged gift to medical staff while mumbling greetings. Often, they would simply leave the envelope or the gift on the doctor's desk without further comments or gesticulation. Medical staff rarely acknowledge the receipt of "the attention."[5] The Romanian context mirrors what Michele Rivkin-Fish described in post-Soviet Russia, where doctors "viewed the failure of the state to provide the necessary resources for public health—to fulfill its basic obligations—as the foundation of corruption and a reasonable justification for bypassing the laws to accept unofficial payments" (2005, 191).

Women from Delcel insisted that, even if different from traditional offerings, the new forms of under-the-table contributions nevertheless signaled the same intention to create personal rapport and elicit attention. Traditional gift offerings confirmed and reinforced a prior connection of mutual reliance, while informal contributions were meant to initiate that relationship. Whether traditional or transformed, offerings to medical staff are intimately linked to time unfolding. Recall that Ana and Crina disagreed about the temporal sequence of offering informal contributions, but they both recognized time as an important variable in defining the nature of interactions surrounding these contributions. Bourdieu shows that "the lapse of time that separates the gift from the counter-gift" (1990, 105) can mask the raw economic exchange between two parties. The distinction between a bribe and gratitude gift can be based on the moment when they take place in the temporal sequence of the medical encounter. Made before (*ex ante*) consultation, contributions are likely to be understood as a bribe, while made after (*ex post*), they are perceived as gratitude gifts (Gal and McKee 2005). The Deontological Code of Romanian Physicians' College does not make any reference to informal payments versus gratitude gifts.[6] This distinction is acknowledged by the Bulgarian Physicians Union (Balabanova and McKee 2002, 246). Similarly, the Hungarian Medical Chamber's Code of Ethics states that "the expression of gratitude, which accompanies recovery from illness, saving of lives and the birth of a new life is not subject to coercion and is based on free will" provided that "within certain limits gratitude payment is legal and legitimate" (Gal and McKee 2005, 1446). Yet the distinction between ex ante and ex post becomes irrelevant when repeated medical encounters are required, such as for prenatal care. In this case, informal contributions "elicited memories of relationships past and . . . begat the material obligation for future exchange" (Kipnis 1997, 58). Camelia, the twenty-five-year-old medical resident in a Bucharest maternity hospital, elaborates on the importance of timing informal contributions during prenatal care: "The bribe you give at the onset of every monthly checkup is meant to build up your future safety. It is about a certitude—which you don't always have—that when you are in labor, the doctor who followed your pregnancy will be there to assist you. If you keep contributing, he will probably be more likely to attend the delivery."

Camelia pauses for a moment before adding with an ironic smile: "Unless the doctor is on vacation, or maybe he does not feel like coming, or maybe he has something else to do." As Camelia pointed out, "the bribe" is an investment in future life, an almost oracular device that mitigates reproductive uncertainty in ways not unlike the traditional bread, soap, and towel offerings. However, successful reproduction remains conditional. No matter how consistent, under-the-table contributions cannot absolutely grant assistance at birth. The OB-GYN's discretionary power (of choosing whether to show up) reinforces people's perceived need for informal payments.

Under-the-table contributions are means to alleviate reproduction-related anxieties, as Ramona's case illustrates. She was one of the women struggling with infertility, first introduced in chapter 1. She gave birth in the mid-1980s to a premature baby girl weighing only 4 pounds who received an Apgar score of 7 and was placed in an incubator for about three weeks. Worried about the fragility of her baby, Ramona recalls making extensive use of informal contributions to the neonatal medical staff:

I gave the nurse way above the average, in both gifts and money, because my daughter was so tiny and I wanted her to receive good care. The nurse would bring the baby from the NICU to me several times a day, just for breastfeeding. I did not see my daughter for the rest of the time. So, to make sure that they would take care of her, that they wouldn't place her under a window or something ... I knew what the average [informal contribution] was and I gave the nurse above that.

Given the economic shortages of the 1980s, Ramona had strategically amassed commodities starting with her college years, with the expectation that her ability to contribute under-the-table would secure her and her baby a better birthing experience: "In college I had foreign classmates who sold things on the underground market. So I made a stock, just in case. I bought soaps. I had *Fa*— that soap was sought for back then. I had deodorants and perfumes. I used the whole stock while in the hospital with my premature baby. It was helpful, because I balanced money payments with gifts. This was the best way to manage the maternity hospital [experience]."

Ramona's account provides another glimpse into the reproductive struggles of women during the late communist era. Suddenly commodified, ordinary western goods circulated through informal exchanges aimed at mitigating women's perceived reproductive vulnerability. Ramona and others acknowledged that informal contributions were bound by the unwritten rules of reciprocity. Giving too little or too much is a faux pas that can cause inadequate forms of care. Yet, Ramona deliberately forced the balanced exchange by contributing more than customarily expected. Anxious about her newborn's fragility, she escalated the magnitude and frequency of informal contributions with the understanding that the medical staff would reciprocate accordingly. Her newborn was eventually dismissed from the NICU. To Ramona, this was evidence not only of the quality of neonatal intensive care but also of the effectiveness of informal contributions to protect future life. Seen through Ramona's eyes, we understand the Delcel women's rationale for linking corruption to reproduction in their comments about the Bucur and Giuleşti incidents. To them, the implication was that, had parturient mothers made consistent informal contributions to Giuleşti NICU staff, the section would not have been left unattended for so long.

As suggested by women's stories and opinions, informal contributions in the field of reproductive care are tactics that both reinscribe and transgress corruption. Naturalized as everyday practice, they nevertheless are perceived as illicit. When acknowledged as ways to exert agency, informal contributions reveal how women reduce perceived reproductive vulnerability and negotiate personhood. In some cases, bribery has the power to protect new life and ensure successful reproduction. More importantly, the prevalence of informal payments in the field of reproductive care sets up women's expectations even when it comes to cervical cancer prevention. Based on their experience with informal contributions for giving birth, the Roma women from Cluj interviewed by Trude Andreassen and her colleagues (2017) avoided free cervical cancer screening provided through a mobile clinic because of the assumption that they would have to contribute under-the-table. As I show in the following section, women from Delcel also viewed informal contributions as crucial in conceptualizing access to forms of reproductive care beyond giving birth.

THE MEDICAL ENCOUNTER

From my conversations with the women who shared their reproductive life histories with me, the medical encounter emerged as a codified mutual exploration between patients and doctors. "To codify" involves normalization and structure (Kaneff 2002, 92), and under-the-table contributions provide both patients and medical staff with predictable mutual interactions. Drawing on Veronica's opinions and Xenia's story, I consider the ways in which informal contributions bound patients and doctors together in ways that obscure the power struggles of the medical encounter (Ferzacca 2000; Trnka 2007). As Rivkin-Fish shows, in Sankt Petersburg maternity hospitals, the expected gender solidarity between women obstetricians and their patients is replaced with "power, domination, inequality, and disenfranchisement [that] traversed multiple and contradictory channels, even when the structure of relations in the clinic clearly favored medical expertise" (2005, 129). However, Rivkin-Fish also cautions against seeing the medical encounter as a mere "binary opposition between powerful doctors and victimized patients" (2005, 22). Informal contributions are an instrument to assert power and tame uncertainty on both sides.

Veronica is one of the most unassuming and solicitous women among those I met in Roşiorii. She looks older than her fifty years because of a slow, limping walk and asthma wheezing. During the 1980s, Veronica was employed as an unskilled heavy industry worker. When the factory closed in the early 1990s, she started doing seasonal work digging gardens or cutting firewood for Delcel families. She usually receives payment in kind. Most people give her food, clothing, or used household articles in exchange for her labor. A victim of domestic violence, Veronica has been the subject of local gossip. And, like other women of Delcel, she had repeated abortions to control her fertility. Her only daughter is married and has one child.

Echoing other women's opinions, Veronica explains the role of informal contributions to ease clinical encounter interactions and reproductive vulnerability: "People give. People give, and you give a small attention. Then you expect the doctor to take a closer look at you or to give birth faster or easier because of this attention." Asked about the temporality of "giving," Veronica opines: "Before [the consultation], before, when you place it in the [doctor's] pocket or leave it on the table. You put it in his pocket, and you say, *Doctor, sir, help me give birth faster and easier.*" Veronica elaborates on instances of patients' satisfaction about the doctor who assists one during delivery:

> To be pleased with your doctor . . . if he comes to see how you are, to ask you how it was, whether you feel fine, whether the baby is fine. Unhappy means that he doesn't come, means that you didn't give him enough and he is uninterested in coming to check on you, uninterested in coming and telling you, *Mommy, how are you? How is your baby doing?* If he doesn't come, that means he is not pleased with how much you have given him; he is not happy with what you have given. Those who are pleased come and say, *Look, the baby is doing this and that. How are you?*

Veronica's description of a typical interaction between a post-parturient mother and her OB-GYN contains coded language and gesticulation that she deciphers for me. Although I elicited from her the definition of a patient's (dis)satisfaction, Veronica eventually twisted her answer and focused instead on the doctor. The patient's satisfaction is conditioned by the doctor's happiness. According to her, a "happy" doctor would provide the attention elicited through the informal contribution to the mother and her newborn. In contrast, an "unhappy" doctor would deliberately withhold attention to show his dissatisfaction with the gift or the lack thereof. As with Ramona's premature baby, the quality of care women receive encodes for patients a feedback communication about the success of their informal contributions to medical staff. Along with the doctor's professional reputation, his quotation on the market of informal contributions played a role in Veronica choosing him to assist with her grandchild's birth: "I heard from other people. They said they gave birth with that one, and [that] he was better than the other one. Also, that one requires as much [informal payment] or maybe it requires as much if you need a C-section. You ask around how much that doctor would take for a normal birth, how much for a C-section . . . and then you chose the cheaper one, if you cannot afford another one. This is how we did it."

While it is difficult to assess all the factors involved in a successful medical encounter, the following tragicomic narrative that circulates in Delcel illustrates what happens when the reciprocity established through informal contributions is violated on one side. With slight variations, I heard this urban legend from four different although not necessarily independent sources. All women who told me this story claimed to have been personally acquainted with the main character, whom I will call Xenia. I met neither Xenia nor her doctor, and I have no evidence that the story is real. She had allegedly moved to Italy a few months before the start of my research.

A longtime Delcel resident in her early fifties, Xenia had decided in the spring of 2007 to have a gynecological exam at the local municipal hospital after feeling a bloating sensation in her lower abdomen for weeks. She went to the hospital, but she stepped into the consultation room without making any informal contributions. She later claimed that she had prepared a gratitude gift to offer once the consultation was over, but she was so perplexed by the diagnosis that she forgot about it. After performing a cursory ultrasound examination, the doctor diagnosed her with uterine cancer. The tumor was large, and Xenia needed urgent surgery. The doctor said he would perform the surgery provided that Xenia made a substantial informal payment of a few hundred euro. Xenia was incredulous. She had only feared pregnancy. She had missed her period for several months and felt some kicks in her belly. Annoyed and pointing to the blurry image of the ultrasound screen, the doctor insisted that she had cancer. She was missing her periods because of menopause, a normal physiological state for her age—he stated. The tumor, however, needed to be removed as soon as she could make the informal contribution. Xenia's family did not have the kind of money the doctor had asked for. As a consequence, one of her daughters went to Italy for a couple of months and worked as a janitor to earn the necessary euro. Upon the daughter's return, the informal payment was made and the surgery date was set. The evening before the scheduled surgery, Xenia and her extended family were sharing one last dinner together when her water broke. Less than two hours later, Xenia had a healthy baby girl, born to term. The story ends on a humorous note. Months later, Xenia is swinging her baby on the porch. To mislead the innocent bypassers, she addresses the baby as a grandmother would talk to her grandchild: "Who's your grandma? Come to grandma!"

The value of this story is that it provides an insight into how people from Delcel understand the role of informal payments in navigating a successful medical encounter. Xenia's case can substantiate our knowledge about the moralities of reproductive care. The story is rather ambiguous.[7] We are left wondering whether the doctor was incompetent (and really thought Xenia had a tumor), whether he purposefully misled his patient (pretending that the fetus was a tumor), or whether he paid so little attention to her symptoms because she had not contributed informally before the consultation. (It is unclear whether the family ever got their money back.)

To the women who recounted it, this narrative was a fable with a moral. Maria and Ileana were the first to tell me Xenia's story together, taking turns, adding details to each other's account and animating voices: "But, doctor, whatever it is in my belly . . . it kicks!" "No, lady, you have a big tumor right in your uterus!" According to Maria and Ileana, the baby was born because Xenia and her family had no money to bribe the doctor and to receive his full attention. Although the doctor made a serious medical error, neither Maria and Ileana, nor the other women who told me the story, raised questions of his professional competence. To them, Xenia's initial failure to contribute under-the-table triggered all that followed. Her transgression set the ground for a dysfunctional medical encounter. The storytellers believed that had she offered an adequate informal contribution, the doctor would have paid attention and would probably have made a different diagnosis. Xenia's failure to pay set up an ambiguous ending because late maternities are seen as an economic burden and a source of social shame. For the women of Delcel, this tale also illustrated the asymmetry of power in the clinical context and the role of informal contributions to restore some power balance. When Xenia discussed her symptoms with the doctor, he promptly rejected them. As long as he was not offered a gift, he barricaded himself behind medico-technological expertise.

The role of humor in this story is important. As Zerilli observed, "Making jokes about corruption is commonplace in today's Romania, a discursive practice in which many persons appear to be involved daily" (2005, 84). People inject humor in their commentaries about the corrupt system in which they are forced to participate. By poking fun at the doctor and making him look like a fool, they effectively knock the medical elite from their pedestals. In this case, humor hints at the fact that doctors are humans with foibles. There is something grotesque about an expert allegedly mistaking a pregnancy for cancer that is captured through "animating voices" (Besnier 2009). Long after listening to the women who recounted this story, the patient's and the doctor's voices still reverberate in my head. It is through ventriloquism that this gossip makes bearable a situation of perceived vulnerability. The story captures the workings of corruption, which prevents medicine from being adequately distributed and cervical cancer prevention from becoming morally justified.

... AS OVERHEARD IN RUMORS

Xenia's story circulates in the Delcel community as a gossip-flavored urban legend. Allegations about dysfunctional reproductive care are prevalent and are expressed through a variety of fluid discursive genres, especially through rumors. In their responses to the HPV vaccination campaign that targeted their prepubescent daughters and granddaughters, some mothers and grandmothers linked apparently disconnected topics, such as mistrust in state-provided reproductive care and apprehensions about additive-laden foods, radioactivity, and environmental pollution. Although variable, their discourses explored the broader themes of reproductive purity and corruption. Corrupted purity was a key assertion in the narratives of Delcel parents when explaining HPV vaccination refusal. Parental narratives tended to be organized into "clusters of rumors" (Campion-Vincent and Scheper-Hughes 2001) that staged corruption as literally embodied—through ingestion, consumption, contact, or injection—into girls' pristine bodies. As Luise White shows, rumors link "the politics of representation" with actual politics, as they "simultaneously reveal popular conceptions about the actions and ideas of those in authority and declare the weakness of official channels of information and education" (1995, 220).

In this section, I look at the multiplicity of entangled rumors concerning reproduction, corruption, and the state. The shifting discourses exploring purity and corruption—through which some parents conveyed anxieties about their daughters being targeted for the vaccine—place a particular twist on the Romanian case of resisting HPV vaccination.

Recall Ana's birthing story from chapter 4. In answer to my question about her reasons for not vaccinating her twelve-year-old daughter against HPV, Ana evoked her skipping both prenatal and postnatal care, reminding me of her long-held mistrust of public reproductive care, whose most recent occurrence was the HPV vaccine. After criticizing the vaccination campaign, Ana suddenly changed the topic to the consumption of additive-laden foods: "All that food they advertise on TV is full of additives [E-uri].[8] But you know what? Even the tomatoes, the potatoes . . . all these are loaded with Es. What are we supposed to eat? We have no choice, don't you see? We are stuffed with chemicals, with poison."

Ana implied that both the HPV vaccine and chemically loaded foods could corrupt young, vulnerable bodies. Hearing Ana, I realized that early during my stay in Delcel, Adriana had handed me a small paper bag with half a dozen eggs freshly gathered from her hens. Adriana had told me that the eggs would be a very healthy choice for my young son because her hens were on an organic corn diet. I understood the special value of Adriana's gift only after repeatedly listening to the Delcel residents' concerns about chemically laden foods and their harmful effects on children.

Ana was not the only one who clustered, in one single narrative, her mistrust of the HPV vaccine with rumors about additive-laden foods. Tereza also drew an explicit parallel between failed state medicine, contaminated food, and corrupted bodies. Although her university education set her apart from most of her neighbors, as a fifty-seven-year-old retired engineer, Tereza was living like many of them, in a small but tidy house with a garden, a pigsty, and some chicken coops. She was long-divorced and had a daughter established in Bucharest. During her discursive exploration of purity and corruption—part of her HPV vaccine criticism—Tereza introduced a new theme: maternal breast milk, which she considered "the only pure and powerful food." At first glance, breast milk seemed to bear little connection to the topic of the HPV vaccine. However, as Jennifer Reich demonstrates in the U.S. context, "Public health claims of the naturalness of breastfeeding may actually increase perceptions of vaccines as unnatural in contrast to breastfeeding, leading to greater distrust of vaccines" (2016, 105). Besides Tereza, other women too backed up their HPV vaccination refusal narratives with reflections about maternal milk and infant formula. According to them, through breastfeeding, a mother preserves the purity of her child. While urging me to not wean my own baby girl too early, Maria contrasted a "corrupted" baby (i.e., prematurely weaned) with a "normal" one (i.e., breastfed until two years of age). "Don't wean her, or you will corrupt the baby! [*Să n-o înţarci, că strici copilu'!*] Do you have to resume work? You can go to your workplace without having to wean her. . . . You return from work in the evening and you breastfeed your baby until she turns two. . . . Hey, that's a normal baby, [made] from breast! [*Copil normal, domnule, din ţâţă.*] No bottle at all!"

Although in their discourses they valued breastfeeding and endorsed maternal milk as pure and powerful, most of the mothers who shared their reproductive life histories with me decided at some point to administer powdered milk to their infants. Most of these mothers made these nutritional decisions for their babies not so much because of practical barriers to breastfeeding—like the need to resume work that Maria mentioned—but rather because of interwoven anxieties and aspirations. On the one hand, they expressed concerns about self-perceived "insufficient" or "poor" breast milk, which they saw as a consequence of their own poor diet. The fluctuating availability of adequate foods (such as meat and fresh fruits) would translate to a mother's "watery milk" (*lapte apăcios*), a type of maternal milk allegedly not suitable for an infant's nutritional needs. Powdered milk appeared as an unchanging and thus reliable source of nutrients, in contrast not only to breast milk but also to other alternatives to breast milk, such as fresh cow's or goat's milk. On the other hand, they regarded infant formula as a coveted market commodity. The commodity value of powdered milk can be traced back to before 1989, when infant formula was available only on the black market through informal connections. Especially western European or U.S. imported brands epitomized technological advancement and capitalist consumption. Feeding the baby with formula equated with an implicit critique of the communist regime. In contrast with mother's milk, which is only biological, powdered milk was invested with symbolic capital through its transmission as a commodity (see also Scheper-Hughes 1992).

After 1989, the sudden visibility of powdered milk on the free market did not strip it of its value as a coveted good. Quite the contrary. Delcel residents' commentaries suggested that, given its high price compared to the buying power of average Romanians, powdered milk reentered the circuit of commodities as an indicator of status consumption. Pharmaceutical representatives aggressively market infant formula and provide family doctors with free samples. Receiving a free can of powdered milk feeds the consumerist aspirations of those mothers who feel otherwise excluded from participation in the market economy. Thirty-two-year-old Sara, mother to two toddlers, recalled her experiences: "Here we often receive it [infant formula] free of charge from the family doctor, until the baby turns one. Not every month, though. But the months when you get it you are happy." Asked why she was feeling happy, Sara continues: "Because you can also give your baby the canned milk, like other mothers do. They can afford to buy it. They go to the supermarket and get it. It's as simple as that!"

Questions arise about parents' contradictory attitudes regarding their children's exposure to what they perceived as potentially harmful biomedical practices. The women from Delcel regarded both the HPV vaccine and powdered milk as potentially soiling in relation to their children's purity. However, while they were adamant that they would prevent their daughters from receiving the HPV vaccine, they did not withhold their infants from the pharmaceutically produced powdered milk. The perceived social status gained by the ability to use infant formula outweighs any fears of the commercial product's corruptive effects on the body. Delcel residents' decision-making flexibility demonstrates that local definitions of purity and corruption are contingent on people's experiences of the state and expectations about the market.

Along with food discourses, ecological themes illustrate citizens' anxieties about society at large (Wilson 2010). Delcel residents' HPV vaccination narratives drew consistently on rumors about endangered reproduction because of radioactive exposure caused by the 1986 Chernobyl nuclear plant disaster. Because of its geographical proximity to Ukraine, Romania experienced high levels of ionizing radiation from the nuclear plant. In addition, the official propaganda channels on both the Soviet and the Romanian sides initially concealed the accident, which increased exposure to harmful radioactivity.

In July 2002, I had already heard Chernobyl tales during a twenty-four-hour stay in a public maternity hospital in Cluj. I shared the room with six other women, all diagnosed with "high-risk pregnancies." As they struggled to make sense of their unexpected state of reproductive vulnerability, they speculated on Chernobyl-related radioactive contamination as a possible factor that triggered their condition. Accidental radiation exposure provided them with a plausible etiology of their state. It also limited their moral responsibility for what some of them perceived as personal reproductive failure. They anchored the deteriorating condition of their bodies in a recent history that was beyond individual control. The corrupted purity of the pregnant body became a link between past, present, and future.

Later, while doing fieldwork in Roșiorii de Vede, I unexpectedly encountered references to the Chernobyl disaster. Some women from Delcel expressed their perceived reproductive vulnerability by discursively shifting back and forth between the HPV vaccine and the Chernobyl accident. The popular belief that women's and men's reproduction has been affected by radioactive contamination is relatively widespread in eastern European countries, including Ukraine (Petryna 2003; Philips 2002), Bulgaria (Kaneff 2002), and Hungary (Harper 2001). Public health reports about the reproductive consequences of exposure to Chernobyl radiation are contradictory.[9] However, it appears that even some obstetricians use Chernobyl rumors in their professional narratives when they are unable to provide a biomedical rationale for painful reproductive events such as miscarriages or infant deaths (Kaneff 2002). The HPV vaccination campaign had activated Delcel residents' perceived sense of reproductive vulnerability. This is why they referred to the Chernobyl accident as a credible explanation for the increase in reproductive problems, such as high rates of infertility in women, miscarriages, and congenital defects. Whether by personal experience or by exposure to mass media reports, people clustered once again in their narratives two different sets of rumors (regarding the HPV vaccine and the Chernobyl disaster, respectively). They explicitly drew a parallel between the communist state failure to protect its citizens from harmful nuclear radiation exposure and the postcommunist state's ineffectiveness to preserve the young girls' purity. In their views, radioactive irradiation and HPV vaccination were intimately linked through their potential of inoculating de facto corruption into the body. In the context of the HPV vaccination debate, the lingering specter of Chernobyl allegations provided a meaningful precedent to highlight the harmful potential that biopolitical experiments gone out of control have on women's reproductive bodies.

CORRUPTION, REPRODUCTION, AND PRISTINE BODIES

The HPV vaccine made some parents uneasy in ways that no other vaccine did. Recall Amalia's fierce rejection of the HPV vaccine as mentioned in chapter 3: "I won't accept this vaccine for my girl. As long as she is a virgin, I will not take any action." Amalia's daughter, twelve-year-old Tina, had been included in the national program's population to receive, free of charge, the three doses of HPV vaccine meant to protect her from the risk of developing cervical cancer later in her life. Amalia's angry outburst did not reflect the ordinary kind of vaccination anxieties expressed by parents worldwide about the pertussis, measles, rubella, or polio vaccines (Feldman-Savelsberg, Ndonko, and Schmidt-Ehry 2000; Bazylevych 2011; Masquelier 2012; Heller 2008; Leach and Fairhead 2007). Like this young mother from Roșiorii de Vede, many other Romanian parents have declined HPV immunization for their daughters on the grounds of the vaccine's potential to corrupt the purity of prepubescent bodies.

As I have shown previously, as they struggled to convey their HPV vaccination anxieties, women from Delcel made use of shifting discourses that explored and redefined the moralities of reproductive care. Like Amalia, other parents referred to their daughters' chaste bodies. Such virginal bodies were seen as constantly exposed to corruption through a wide range of potentially polluting actions, including the inoculation of biological material through vaccination. What Amalia feared was not that the vaccine would prompt Tina to prematurely start her sexual life and become exposed to sexually transmitted infections (STIs). Amalia referred to Tina's virginal condition in a broader sense, to convey her daughter's purity. Like many other Romanian parents and grandparents, Amalia did not see her daughter "at risk" for cervical cancer. Her main concern was to preserve the pristine state of her child. Maria expressed a similar preoccupation for withholding children from potentially disrupting medical intervention. When I first asked her about the HPV vaccine, she snapped at me: "Mind your own business! What vaccine? Do not accept any vaccine! You should not give drugs to children!"

Cross-culturally, preteenagers are culturally and socially liminal beings. Their genderless anatomies do not bear childhood traits anymore, but they only promise future sexuality and reproductive potential. Because of their structural and symbolic ambiguity, prepubescent bodies epitomize local ideas about purity and danger, pollution and taboo, norm and transgression, which become manifest in social, political, and cultural constructions of feminine sexuality (Bernau 2007; Douglas 1969). Gail Kligman shows that in much of rural and peri-urban Romania, "virginity and purity are fetishized and sacralized. . . . Complex beliefs about pollution, honor, virginity, and shame have been constructed in cultural self-defense against the physical manifestation of female maturity" (1988, 67). There are specific funeral rituals for virgins, proximity taboos for menstruating young women, and metaphors that refer to pubescent girls as "blossoming forth" and to menarche as "flowers on one's skirt."

The topic of the virginal female body came up repeatedly in conversations about HPV vaccination anxieties. The women who spoke with me actively imagined the grandchildren they will possibly have. Yet they found it distressing to think of their prepubescent daughters as actively sexual and prone to STIs, as the HPV campaign suggested. The standard medical protocol is to administer vaccines as early as possible to minimize the risk of exposure. But since HPV is transmitted mainly through genital contact, the targeting of prepubescent girls by health authorities was disturbing to parents. To evoke the possibility of STIs in the lives of young girls was to deny them the innocence they embodied. To some parents, the act of vaccination even came to equate a symbolic defloration. Through their vaccination, these girls become defined as sexual subjects. Thus, in resisting the vaccine, the parents were also resisting the potential subjectification of their daughters as sexual beings. Alina is a stay-at-home wife and mother of Bianca (age 14), Anca (age 11), and Teo (age 6). Referring to the school medical nurses who were supposed to administer the vaccine to her older daughter, Alina rhetorically asked: "How could I allow *them* to take over my child? If something would happen to her [because of the vaccine] wouldn't I be to blame? But if not [vaccinated] and she gets ill later, do you think she would blame me for [her illness]?" Given the pristine condition of their daughters' healthy bodies, immunization appeared threatening to Amalia and Alina. These mothers redefined preventive care as withholding their daughters from the circulation of global biomedical (and, by extension, moral) values. A parent's duty was to preserve a child's purity. We have, nevertheless, to acknowledge that Alina seems to be torn between accepting and refusing the vaccine. Her ambivalent attitude is illustrative for the kind of dilemmas parents were facing when considering the

HPV vaccination for their daughters. Some people were concerned that under the guise of protecting girls' reproductive health, the state was once again reaching too far in the private lives of its citizens.

CONCLUSIONS

Corruption looms large in the moral imagination of Romanians. Narratives of corruption—fed by mass media accounts—establish a conceptual frame that justifies the use of informal connections and contributions. In the field of reproductive care, informal contributions are not only responses to perceived reproductive vulnerability. They are personalizing, savvy tactics of participation in a culture of supply-and-demand that preceded, temporally and symbolically, the market economy. This moral economy of gifts—encapsulated within a market economy—brings about new claims and entitlements.

Delcel residents' shifting discourses about the moralities of reproductive care staged a parallelism between the individual body, social body, and body politics. "When the sense of social order is threatened . . . there is a strong concern with matters of ritual and sexual purity, often expressed in vigilance over social and bodily boundaries" (Scheper-Hughes and Lock 1987, 24). In Delcel women's narratives surrounding the delivery of reproductive care, corruption intersects all three bodies. When it refers to illicit or fraudulent interactions and procedures, corruption is, after all, a metaphor that stands for a dysfunctional social body and body politics. However, when it comes to prepubescent girls, corruption has the threatening potential of being literally inoculated into individual bodies through vaccination. People used their stories of reproductive vulnerability and embodied corruption to justify the withholding of young female bodies from mainstream medical discourses and practices. The ideas about corrupted purity expressed in relation to the HPV vaccine, while articulated at multiple discursive levels, become part of an attempt to "purify" both the social and the individual body.

The ubiquitous preoccupation with the moralities of reproductive care in general, and the parental concerns about what is being injected into their daughters' pristine bodies in particular, are responses to the uncertainties surrounding state and private medicine transformations that I explored in chapters 4 and 5. Cervical cancer prevention programs activated Romanians' concerns about the ethics of care and provided people with a platform to express their conflicting views of post-communist medicine. Because it is embedded in neoliberal reforms—which are themselves sites of corruption and alienation—cervical cancer prevention has failed to become a source of authoritative knowledge.

CONCLUSION
The Space between Informed and Non-Informed Refusal

In accounting for the historical, political, and cultural circumstances of reproductive health care and cervical cancer prevention in contemporary Romania, I have deliberately chosen history as the point of entry. A repressive recent history of state control over reproduction has had ripple effects. Traumatic experiences generated by past reproductive policies have resurfaced during current government and nongovernmental attempts to manage the sexual and reproductive health of Romanian women, old and young. Decades after the end of the communist pronatalism, Romanian women still mistrust medical interventions aimed at female reproductive bodies.

But reproduction is more than just about individuals. Patriarchal ideas and practices shaming women's sexuality while celebrating motherhood have shaped local understandings of reproductive health and health care even before the pronatalist era. Socialized into forms of everyday patriarchy, women of southern rural and peri-urban Romania perceive domestic violence as unavoidable, abortion as the sole means of birth control, gynecological exams as embarrassing, sexually transmitted infections (STIs) as the result of promiscuous behavior, and menopause as granting one an exemption from preventive care. Men and boys retain the privilege of staying invisible from the realm of reproduction not only in everyday life but also in health promotion and prevention. Even though men also get infected, in contemporary Romania, the human papillomavirus (HPV) is seen exclusively as a woman's burden.

With receiving unreliable reproductive support from either the state or their male partners, some women articulate HPV vaccination refusal on behalf of their daughters or granddaughters through lived religion narratives. To them, God's will has an ontological correlate in embodied reproductive experiences, from conception and abortion to birth and gynecologic cancers. By delegating future reproductive health to God, women attempt to solve a moral dilemma:

Leave girls unvaccinated (and therefore untouched and pristine) now, but expose them to presumed future illness, or vaccinate them now (and, thus, tamper with their pure bodies) in exchange for the promise of undamaged health. Lived religion also normalizes abortion as a redeemable everyday practice. This may be consequential to women's health, given the still controversial link between repeated abortions and an increase in cervical cancer risk.

Fashioned by patriarchal relations, lived religion, and the historical trauma of pronatalism, women's responses to reproductive health care and cervical cancer prevention have been complicated by postcommunist reforms to medical care. Romanians have had to contemplate the idea that their health may no longer be defined solely by the state. Increasingly exposed to models of care that redefine sexual and reproductive health as a commodity with monetary value, women struggle to reimagine personhood somewhere beyond both a weakened state and a merciless liberalized market. When preventive screening, managed by nongovernmental organizations (NGOs), occupied that interstitial space between state and private medicine, women would nevertheless decline free health care services. Rather than actively seeking care through the existing channels of cervical cancer prevention, they would choose to only engage with the moralities of reproductive medicine. Women's narratives of purity and corruption connect the individual, the market and the state.[1] By activating people's counternarratives of corruption, cervical cancer prevention—and especially the HPV vaccination campaign—has provided Romanians a legitimate instance to express their conflicting views of postcommunist medical reforms. In the end, women "talk corruption" to validate a more pristine, uncontaminated self, outside of the postcommunist state and the neoliberal market.[2]

The historical and structural forces that I have documented throughout this book in relation to cervical cancer prevention are also at play elsewhere in the world. There are other instances of extreme pronatalist policies, of patriarchal agendas shaping women's sexual and reproductive well-being, and of people invoking nonsecular rationalities to explain their reproductive decision-making. Worldwide, suspicions and accusations of corruption have intensified as countries and communities struggle to reform dysfunctional and unjust medical care systems.

Romania is not the only state that ratified strict pronatalist policies in the past half century. With exceptions to criminalizing abortion (such as endangerment of a woman's life, a physically or mentally disabled woman, congenital malformation of the fetus, incest, and rape), the Romanian pronatalism of the 1966–1989 period was not even the most draconian in recent history. For example, in Ireland, between 2014 and 2019, the only legal ground for an abortion was endangering a woman's life (Erdman 2014). As of 2020, in Poland, the amendment to eliminate the legal right to an abortion in case of severe fetal anomaly is still under consideration in parliament after mass protests. In Argentina, until 2006, surgical birth control methods such as tubal ligation and vasectomy were criminalized (Peñas Defago and Moran Faúndes 2014). However, communist Romania's pronatalist policies were quite unique in at least two ways. First, in Catholic countries such as Ireland, Poland, and Argentina, pronatalist policies were enforced in the name of the sanctity of life from conception (Erdman 2014; Mishtal 2009; Mishtal 2015; Peñas Defago and Moran Faúndes 2014), but the vision behind the Romanian pronatalism was a secular one. Second, and perhaps more important, the communist authorities enforced pronatalism through extreme political surveillance. The policing of reproduction and reproductive health produced long-term individual and transgenerational traumas that, as I argued in chapters 1 and 2, shape women's current mistrust in state reproductive medicine.

Romania is also not exceptional in the frequency with which people would look at women's sexuality and gynecologic cancers through a patriarchal, stigmatizing lens. Dudgeon and Inhorn (2004) reviewed numerous cross-cultural ethnographic examples of men's influence on women's reproductive health, from conception and abortion to STIs, pregnancy, birth, and infertility. Yet, as I showed in chapter 2, through reproductive invisibility rather than open involvement, Romanian men shape women's health and well-being. Romania is also not unique in having women mobilize religion, in either canonical or noncanonical versions, as part of reproductive decision-making. Unlike the Polish Catholic Church that provided secular authorities with the foundational ideology for a "moral governance" (Mishtal 2009, 2015), the Romanian Orthodox Church was unable to fashion a mainstream narrative about the morality of reproduction. But, as I demonstrated in chapter 3, Romanian women have adjusted their Orthodox faith to everyday lived reproductive events, not unlike their Catholic and Evangelical counterparts did in some parts of the United States (McGuire 2008).

Romania is among the postcommunist countries from the eastern bloc and beyond to reform state medicine and to privatize some sectors of health care. Like people in post-Soviet Russia (Rivkin-Fish 2005; Temkina and Rivkin-Fish 2020) and post-Soviet Cuba (Andaya 2014; Brotherton 2012), Romanian women navigate the maze of familiar and strange pathways that make up the emergent landscapes of care. As I showed in chapters 4 through 6, in the face of the dismantling of state medicine, women's engagement with reproductive health care is more tactical than strategic. In Romania, like in Russia (Rivkin-Fish 2005; Ledeneva 2006), Lithuania (Praspaliauskiene 2016), or Cuba (Andaya 2009), informal contributions are understood as crucial in securing access to privileged care. Women's struggles are amplified by the multiplication of channels of medical care distribution brought about by the partial privatization of medicine. Stuck at the crossroad between state-provided and market-driven reproductive health care, some women would choose to withhold their own and their daughters' bodies from any preventive intervention. Like Indian (Towghi 2010),

Canadian (Connell and Hunt 2010), and U.S. parents (McRee et al. 2011; Gottlieb 2018), Romanian mothers have also contested cervical cancer prevention on moral grounds. Some of them have echoed concerns about the sexual and reproductive health and well-being of teenagers that were documented elsewhere, too (Wailoo et al. 2010; Coleman, Levison, and Sangi-Haghpeykar 2011; Sam et al. 2009). As I showed in chapter 6, southern rural Romanian mothers expressed their ambivalence toward the HPV vaccine in particular ways, through clusters of rumors opposing purity to corruption.

Taken separately, pronatalism, patriarchy, lived religion, medical reforms, and moral contestation of preventive medicine are not Romanian phenomena, even if they have a particular local flavor. What sets Romania apart is that these structural forces are aligned in constellations of systemic contingencies that expose cervical cancer's inexorable historical, social, and cultural trajectories.

Speaking to the latencies made manifest by the cervical cancer prevention programs, the book is traversed by a multitude of specters (Derrida [1994] 2006; Good 2020), past and present, some persistent, others just flickering apparitions. The women who lived their reproductive years under communism are still haunted by the traumas of mandatory gynecological exams, while an abortion counseling project law threatens to revive the oppressive ghosts of past demographic policies (chapter 1). Made reproductively invisible by a paternalist communist state now long gone, men have remained shadowy in relation to women's reproduction and reproductive health promotion (chapter 2). In refusing preventive screening and vaccination by invoking God's will, people resist the spectrality of being presymptomatic (chapter 3). The horror evoked by newborns burned to death in a public hospital and the lingering anxieties produced by the Chernobyl disaster make women mistrust a deeply corrupted and ineffective system of state medicine (chapter 6). In accessing present-day public maternity hospitals, women encounter the dreadful, albeit often familiar, specters of hospitals past (chapters 4 through 6), or the shiny ghosts of contemporary private clinics (chapter 5), and occasionally, even the fleeting presence of the well-sanitized western clinics from the European Union (chapter 6). Neither public nor private, the NGO-affiliated mobile clinic is also shrouded in evocative veils that make people—socialized into informal payments or fee-for-service—doubt the existence of adequate free care. Sometimes, specters come to light in liminal moments as gloomy reminders of past personal and historical traumas. Before her life-saving hysterectomy, in a hallucination that makes her dread the surgery for a moment, Oana feels the presence of the enigmatic individual who policed her reproductive body decades ago (chapter 1). Maria's attempts to imagine the afterlife are troubled by an eerie vision of her aborted fetuses (chapter 3). Long after Xenia has moved abroad, Maria, Ileana, and other women are still haunted by her grotesque story of reproductive vulnerability that delegitimizes, in their view, the authoritative knowledge of preventive medicine (chapter 6). Finally, Oana's grandfather coming back from forced labor emerges from the dark as an emaciated ghostly image of his old self—an actual embodiment of being subjected to political oppression (chapter 1).

In the light of historical latencies and systemic contingencies, what is the value of this ethnography of reproductive health care and cervical cancer prevention? In this book, I have chronicled Romania's cervical cancer prevention campaigns as "failures foretold." I have highlighted some of the spots where both the Health Ministry and the NGOs missed the mark with generic and inadequate approaches to screening and vaccination promotion and delivery. Western anthropologists familiar with the Romanian medical system have noted the health care officials' "double talk" and have raised questions about their reformist intentions (Kideckel 2008; Friedman 2009; Stillo 2011; O'Neill 2017). The repeated and increasingly downgraded attempts to promote and deliver cervical cancer prevention that I have described in the two interludes suggest that the pathways of medical care delivery remain dysfunctional in contemporary Romania.

From an applied perspective, this book could nevertheless provide health policy makers with a culturally sensitive insight for future attempts to redesign cervical cancer prevention for those who need it the most—the Romanian women from rural, remote, and underserved areas. One of my intentions in writing an ethnography such as this was to "capture the rich variety and texture of life" (Heller 2019,199), to the benefit of public health experts and medical providers. The series of systemic contingencies that I have examined in *The Cancer Within* provide us not only with a lens to understand Romania's puzzling cervical cancer statistics, but also with a tool to imagine future public health solutions. Since they reflect historically articulated structural forces, systemic contingencies are hard to dismantle. Romanian women's lives and reproductive well-being will continue to be shaped by reproductive policies, patriarchal ideology and practice, (non)secular understandings of risk and prevention, medical care reforms, allegations of corruption, and informal circuits of reciprocity.

However, some of the contingencies that these structural forces expose could be reassigned to ensure more successful ways of providing medical care. Based on the ethnographic findings presented in this book, I envision here two specific strategies (beyond the more obvious effort to educate people about HPV and cervical cancer, using health promotion materials that would at least feature actual local women and girls). The first strategy derives from the importance of history—as both remembering the past and imagining the future—in shaping Romanian women's reproductive bodies and lives. As I have demonstrated throughout this book, the historical trauma of the communist pronatalism has left enduring effects that impact some women's willingness to participate in various reproductive health care programs, including cervical cancer prevention. While there is little that can be done to alleviate the suffering of the past, imagining a better future remains within the realm of possibilities. Cervical cancer prevention could be redesigned to provide women with a more robust sense of what the future might bring. More specifically, I suggest enrolling women in a coherent, rigorous program of follow-up gynecological exams at the time of an initial Pap test. This would allow women to see reproductive care as an integral part of their own lives unfolding toward a hopeful future, rather than perceiving a Pap test as a random, inconsequential examination, more akin to the reproductive surveillance of the communist past. The second strategy grows from understanding the scope of the vulnerabilities created by patriarchal ideology and practice, not only for women but also for men. Following the example of the United States, the United Kingdom, Australia, and other countries, I suggest vaccinating boys against the human papillomavirus alongside girls. This could help break the vicious circle of men's reproductive invisibility that I have examined in this book. These suggested solutions to rethink cervical cancer prevention may improve the overall health and well-being for the next generation of Romanian women and men.

When twenty-nine-year-old Ana boasted, in chapter 4, about skipping both prenatal and postnatal care, she also confided: "Even if they burned me alive, I wouldn't willingly go to a gynecologist" [*Nu m-aş duce de bună voie la ginecolog, nici arsă*]. Then she laughed, maybe realizing that her words were dramatic. I looked at her, wondering why a high school–educated mother of two, who was still a child when the communist pronatalism ended, would make such a statement. Did she mean it, or was this just a way of talking? What was she trying to convey? Historical and cultural contingencies aside, how different is Ana from, for instance, an anti-vaccination school parent in California (Sobo 2015) or a pro-gun mother of a teen who committed gun suicide in Missouri (Metzl 2019)? As anthropologists, we are reminded that people are more than just calculated, economic players who act in ways that could unambiguously be perceived as serving their own self-interest. Throughout this book, I have shown that while most women understood the causal link between HPV and cervical cancer, and between Pap screening and cervical cancer early detection, they still chose not to enroll in preventive care. What they dismissed was not the link itself but its relevance to their lives. Women privileged one set of rationalities over another. Medical experts would typically cast such attitudes as "non-informed refusal" of medical intervention (Berlinger and Jost 2010). But, as I have demonstrated, women's culturally and historically situated rationalities both accommodate and resist normative health prevention discourses. Romanian women reserve the right to define "self-interest" in their own terms. They choose to occupy the space between informed and non-informed refusal.

ACKNOWLEDGMENTS

This book project started as a doctoral dissertation during my time at Tulane University in New Orleans. My deepest gratitude goes to Adeline Masquelier, whose mentorship allowed me to grow, through trial and error, into the anthropologist I am today. Adeline taught me to complicate without obscuring and to streamline without essentializing. I also owe significant thanks to Allison Truitt, who guided me with tact and intelligence and knew when I needed some tough love. I am grateful to several other anthropology faculty from Tulane. A long afternoon chat with Mariana Mora, in her brand-new, still empty office, remains in my memory as a moment of sudden clarity. I was fortunate to have similar illuminating conversations with Bob Hill, Alessandra Bazzano, and João Gonçalves. My pathway to social sciences has also been shaped by encounters with archaeologists and biological anthropologists who I am honored to call my friends. John Verano, Lukáš Friedl, and David Chatelain stirred my interests and kept anthropology wonderfully engaging. I am particularly indebted to Jason Nesbitt, who has read every word I wrote in the last several years and has constantly encouraged me along the way.

If the idea of the book originated during my time as a graduate student, working on the manuscript became an everyday reality while I was a visiting assistant professor at Montana State University (MSU) in Bozeman. One of the most consequential moments in the writing process of this book happened during one snowy evening, in a crowded pizza place next to the MSU campus. With cozy ambient noise in the background, my friend and colleague Jim Meyer improvised a brainstorming session about my book manuscript, in search of a working title that we eventually scribbled on a pink Post-it note. The title bestowed a sudden new reality on the manuscript and boosted my confidence. Since then, Jim has constantly inspired and motivated me to write this book. I also want to recognize and thank other colleagues from MSU who supported and promoted my research: David Cherry, Betsy Danforth, and especially Larry Carucci.

My new colleagues at Creighton University have surrounded me with love and attention and created a supportive environment, allowing me to complete the manuscript. Most notably, my two fellow medical anthropologists, Alex Roedlach and Laura Heinemann, as well as now-emerita Barbara Dilly read and provided useful criticism on parts of the manuscript. I am grateful to them, as well as to Angie Lederach, Renzo Rosales, Erin Blankenship-Sefczek, and Kevin Estep. I am lucky to have also had colleagues and friends from other universities providing useful advice and support at various stages of the book writing process. I would like to thank Marcia Inhorn, Joana Mishtal, Liz Roberts, Sabina

Stan, Eugene Raikhel, and Jonathan Stillo. My appreciation also goes to the participants at several workshops: "Therapeutic Encounters: Emerging Research in Health and Medicine in Eastern Europe" at Indiana University in Bloomington; "Lived Religion in the Black Sea Region" in Kyiv, Ukraine; and the Cascadia Seminar in Medical Anthropology at Western Washington University in Bellingham. My special thanks go to my students from Tulane, Montana State, and Creighton. Throughout the years, many of them inspired and energized me with their thoughtful and genuine curiosity. Having had the privilege to work with them makes me hopeful about the future of the humankind.

I am deeply indebted to the people from Roșiorii de Vede who shared with me their stories and welcomed me into their houses. I thank Marius Benţa, Alina Bârsan, Nicuşor Turcan, and Dr. CT, who provided logistical support and help during my field research. My work in Romania was made possible by the generous financial support from several Tulane Anthropology Department summer merit fellowships and from the Paul and Elizabeth Selley dissertation fellowship. I was also granted a dissertation writing fellowship from Tulane University's Murphy Institute Center for Ethics and Public Affairs. Funding from Creighton University allowed me to wrap up the editing of the book manuscript. Early versions of several paragraphs in the book appeared in *Medical Anthropology Quarterly*, *Medical Anthropology*, *Journal of Religion and Health*, and *Culture, Health and Sexuality*.

At various stages of the book writing, several of my close friends read early drafts, commented, and offered useful advice and editing suggestions. I would like to thank John Wright, Mike Pichik, Allison Groove, and especially Kelly Lewis—my "personified English thesaurus." Greg Merchant provided invaluable assistance with processing the images in the book (and cooked for me several delightful meals). Cristina, Ana, Catherine, Frank, and Father David made my life in Bozeman so full of joy. Rob kept me grounded through endless conversations on biking trails and on the ski lift. My most sincere gratitude goes to all of them.

For someone like me—"on a visa"—the only permanent thing about life in the United States is that it has been provisional for the last seventeen years . . . and counting. When contingencies are perpetual, administrative support literally becomes vital in allowing a life of teaching, research, and writing to continue. I owe a huge debt to a series of visionary women who used their administrative powers and fought through the maze of "alien status" bureaucracy on my behalf: at Tulane University, Victoria Bricker, then-chair of the Anthropology Department; at Montana State University, Kristen Intemann, director of the Women, Gender, and Sexuality Studies program, as well as Ilse-Mari Lee, dean of the Honors College, and Waded Cruzado, the university's president; at Creighton University, Bridget Keegan, dean of the College of Arts and Sciences.

I am thrilled about the opportunity to publish this book at Rutgers University Press in the series "Medical Anthropology: Health, Inequality, and Social Justice."

I am tremendously grateful to Lenore Manderson for her generosity and mentorship. Moving forward, I take with me so much from what Lenore has taught me about becoming a better writer. My heartfelt thanks also go to Kimberly Guinta, who has moved the book through the editorial process in such a graceful and upbeat way, and to the two anonymous reviewers who provided thoughtful suggestions and advice.

Finally, I would like to thank my family—my mother, my brother, my children Pavel and Letiția, and their father. I am truly blessed to have you all on my side.

NOTES

INTRODUCTION

1. I draw here on insights from Farmer (2001) connecting infections to social inequalities and from the critique of the social determinants of health by Chenhall and Senior (2018).

2. In the last decades, the practice of fieldwork has changed from "sharing firsthand the environment, problems, background, language, rituals, and social relations of a more-or-less bounded and specified group of people" (Van Maanen 2011, 3) to anthropologists engaging in multisited ethnography to better account for transnational migration or globalization (Clifford and Marcus 1986).

1 "WE ALL DESCEND FROM COMMUNISM"

1. The "obsessive decade" refers to the 1950s. During the post-Stalinist liberalization of the 1960s and 1970s, an entire generation of Romanian writers obsessively recalled the horrors of the 1950s.

2. As stipulated by Decree 770, abortion was legally available only to women over age 45 or for those who already had four living children. From 1985, the quota was raised to five living children. Other exceptions that granted an abortion were endangerment of mother's life, serious congenital malformation of the fetus, mother's physical or psychological health compromised, incest, and rape (Kligman 1998; Doboş, Jinga, and Soare 2010).

3. Birth rates increased from 14.3 live births per 1,000 population in 1966 to 28 in 1968. Total fertility rates reached 3.7 children per woman in 1968, compared to 1.9 children per woman in 1967 (Kligman 1998).

4. My findings concur with previous accounts about the number of back-alley abortions during the 1970s and 1980s. Out of the forty-three women who shared their reproductive life histories with me, twenty-three bore children before 1989. Twenty of them confessed to having had induced abortions before 1989, ranging in number from two abortions (for eight women) to thirty abortions (one woman). Among these twenty women, the average estimated number of abortions per woman was between seven and eight. Given that approximately ten abortions happened legally before 1966, my findings are similar to the nationwide estimated average number of five abortions per woman of reproductive age (15–44 years) between 1966 and 1989 (Şerbănescu et al. 1995). These statistics provide only a relative idea about the number of clandestine abortions. Memory failure or attempts to conceal the real number of abortions impacted their accuracy. Although it may seem invalid to include the woman who claimed having had the extremely high number of thirty abortions, it is safe to assume that she had at least half the number of abortions she claimed. Among the nine women featured in Kligman (1998), two had five abortions each, one had seven abortions, and another one had sixteen abortions. Băban (1999, 2000) also quotes studies that found a sizable proportion of women who had twenty to thirty abortions.

5. In Cristian Mungiu's 2007 fictional cinematic story of a back-alley abortion gone wrong, *4 Months, 3 Weeks and 2 Days*, the procedure takes place in a hotel room. Although there is no ethnographic evidence of clandestine abortions in hotel rooms, the story is a veridical one.

6. The cost of a clandestine abortion varied between 3,000 and 5,000 lei (Kligman 1998; Iepan 2005). At the 1970s exchange rate, that represents between $671 and $1,118 for an abortion in U.S. dollars. During the 1980s, the cost of an abortion was between $268 and $446.

7. Clandestine abortions led to an increase in maternal mortality, from 0.2 for 100 live births in 1965 to 1.5 for 100 live births in 1983 (Kligman 1998, 214). Unsuccessful abortions could also produce poor birth outcomes and increased infant mortality rates (David and Băban 1996; Kligman 1998; Băban 1999).

8. See "Carlos Galli Mainini," Museum of Contraception and Abortion, https://muvs.org /en/topics/pioneers/carlos-galli-mainini-1914-1961-en/.

9. The high school curricula now include sexual and health education classes. The Ministry of Health and the Ministry of Education launched several national information campaigns about contraception and the transmission and prevention of sexually transmitted infections (STIs), targeting teenagers. Pamphlets and posters were distributed through schools, medical practices, clinics and pubs, and advertisements on broadcast radio and TV.

10. The postcommunist governments have promoted elitist familial policies to increase fertility among those with a high socioeconomic status who usually plan to have fewer children. Law 63/1993 introduced the universal child allowance, distributed through local offices of social protection for children younger than school age and through schools for older children. Only in 2007, the law was modified to allow children who did not attend school to receive the allowance. In 2003, the universal child allowance was supplemented for social cases with a means-tested child allowance. The eligibility threshold was set high, and it has increased every year since its inception so that fewer and fewer children are eligible to receive it. For each birth, parents receive a modicum birth indemnity, but only for the first four children. Paid maternity leave is available only for mothers who were employed and contributed to the public insurance fund for at least twelve months before giving birth. The value of the maternity leave is earning-related, but the maximum amount is capped. Paid maternity leave is available only for three children per woman. Such policies have daunted the most fertile categories of population—including the Roma minority—which are also the poorest.

11. Romanian news agency Mediafax, April 4, 2012, https://www.mediafax.ro/social /societatea-civila-cere-guvernului-sa-respinga-proiectul-de-lege-privind-consilierea-inainte -de-avort-9477177.

12. In order to grant women their right to make informed choices, it is necessary to establish abortion management centers/practices. The centers' mission would be to eliminate the risk of a hasty decision with a definitive outcome, which would negatively impact both the woman in question and the future of the entire nation. (In Romanian in original: *Din aceste motive și pentru a elimina riscul de a lua o decizie pripită, al cărei deznodământ nu mai poate fi schimbat și care are efecte atât asupra femeii respective, cât și asupra viitorului națiunii, se impune ca necesară existența unor centre/cabinete specializate pe problematica avortului, care să asigure dreptul la informare al femeii ce deține puterea de decizie în a alege.*) See *Gândul News*, April 23, 2012, http://www.gandul.info/news/avortul-doar-cu-aviz-de-la-psiholog-pdl-promoveaza-o-lege -care-sa-rezolve-criza-demografica-a-romaniei-9488812.

13. See, for instance, "Neo-decreţeii" ("The New Children of the Decree"), *CriticAtac*, March 30, 2012, http://www.criticatac.ro/15486/15486/.

2   REPRODUCTIVE INVISIBILITY

1. In a restricted sense, patriarchy "refers to . . . the sole control of domestic and public-political authority by senior males within the group" (Seymour-Smith 1986, 217). In practice, however, male monopoly on public discourse often coexists with forms of male-female com-

plementarity. From a distinct perspective, some feminists use patriarchy to refer to male social dominance.

2. Starting with the early 1960s, the number of households with one or two adults and dependent children increased, while the number of households with three or more adults and dependent children decreased (Hărăguș 2014).

3. *Monitorul Oficial* no. 4/27, December 1989. Out of the initial thirty-nine members of the "Frontul Salvării Naționale" (FSN)—the executive political organ of the new regime—only five were women. See the complete list of FSN members at https://ioniliescu.wordpress.com /media/comunicat-catre-tara-al-cfsn-22-dec1989/.

4. Particularly after 2000, the households with three or more adults with dependent children increased, while households with one or two adults and dependent children decreased.

5. All married women who talked to me had taken their husband's family names at marriage. None of them expressed the desire to challenge this custom. One woman considered the bureaucratic advantage of preserving one's maiden name.

6. Daughters represent a triple loss: for the patrilineage, for the household economy, and for a father's social standing. According to Oana, "Almost all men want to have boys. [They want] to replicate their sex, their name, and so on. It is about virility, about manhood; they think they are manlier if they have boys. [*Laughs.*]" Informal discussions with several men (ranging from ages 22 to 78) concurred with Oana's comments and demonstrated a generational continuity in preferring sons over daughters.

7. In Romanian, in original: *Soacră, soacră, poamă acră, / De te-ai coace cât te-ai coace, / Dulce tot nu te-i mai face; / De te-ai coace toată toamna, / Ești mai acră decât coarna.* Translated into English by Ana Cartianu.

8. Translated from Romanian by Ana Cartianu.

9. Romanian has morphological suffixes that mark gender in nouns.

10. Documentary sources about the availability of male contraception and men's willingness to engage in contraception are scarce. Condoms were never formally banned throughout the pronatalist years, but the official supply was intermittent and did not cover the demand. On the black market, condoms were expensive and of poor quality. As of 1987, male surgical sterilization (vasectomy) was strongly discouraged, and it appears, mostly unavailable (Doboș, Jinga, and Soare 2010). Knowledge about male contraception did not improve after 1989. A 1995 reproductive health assessment showed that "male sterilization is nearly unknown, even among health professionals, and often is confused with castration" (Șerbănescu et al. 1995, 85).

11. According to women surveyed in David and Băban (1996), most of their male partners were unwilling or unable to co-participate in contraception. However, unlike most women from Delcel, the women surveyed by David and Băban recognize their husbands as active decision-makers regarding abortion (though not so much involved in the practical steps to secure an abortion for their wives). This difference may be due to the higher level of education of women (and presumably men) in David and Băban's sample.

12. While attending yearly remembrance rituals by my grandmother's grave in 1980s, I noticed, year after year, the mourners at the nearby grave of a twenty-seven-year-old woman—her surviving mother and her young son. I kept wondering for years why she died so young and where her husband was. Years later, my mother told me that the young woman had allegedly died from complications of a clandestine abortion and that, on hearing the news of her dying, the husband had a nervous breakdown and had been hospitalized ever since in a mental health institution.

13. It is difficult to estimate the percentage of women and, respectively, of men who performed clandestine abortions during the Ceaușescu era. Ethnographic and anecdotal evidence suggests

that the OB-GYN who would perform clandestine abortion were mostly men (since more men than women had formal medical training), while the untrained abortion providers tended to be mostly women.

14. Women started to publicly debate reproductive policies only in 2012, in response to the mandatory pre-abortion counseling project law (mentioned in chapter 1).

15. In 2008, Romania had a population of 21,504,442 (Gheorghe 2011).

INTERLUDE (PART 1)

1. See *Cuvantul Ortodox*, http://www.cuvantul-ortodox.ro/recomandari/laurentiu-streza -impotriva-vaccinurilor-anti-hpv-gripei-porcine-video-pastorale-sfantul-nicolae/.

2. Ordinance 1612/2008 stipulated the following: Annex 1 letter A point 15 paragraph (1) introduces new letter h) HPV vaccine, using the funds allotted to the National Oncology program. Annex 2 letter A section II National programs regarding noncommunicable diseases, point 2 National oncology program, subtitle Activities, introduces an additional point 5 "HPV vaccination of girls from 4th grade, to prevent cervical cancer, to be realized in schools, by schools' medical practitioners. Note: refusal to allow vaccination will be made by written declaration of parents, while taking the consequences for refusal." Annex 2 letter A section II National programs regarding noncommunicable diseases, point 2 National oncology program, subtitle Evaluation indicators: "Results indicators: vaccinate the cohort of [girls] 10 years old . . . to prevent cervical cancer. Physical indicators: number of girls vaccinated 110,000, number of vaccine doses 330,000. Efficiency indicators: average cost per vaccine dose—300 lei."

3. Blog post, https://www.petreanu.ro/vaccinul-anti-cancer-bigotii-vs-medicina/.

4. News sources at *Ziare.com* (http://www.ziare.com/vaslui/articole/doze+vaccin+hpv+expi rate) and *Ştirile Pro TV* (http://stirileprotv.ro/stiri/sanatate/cancerul-de-col-uterin-ucide-iar -dozele-de-vaccin-hpv-expira-in-depozite.html).

3   BEYOND RATIONALITIES

1. The Romanian Orthodox Church—Biserica Ortodoxă Română (BOR)—claims the status of "national church." In 2011, out of 19,043,767 Romanians 16,367,267 (that is, 85.94 percent) declared themselves Orthodox Christians (INSSE 2011). After 1989, BOR attempted to claim authority over reproduction, but it failed for at least two reasons. First, from 1948 to 1989, BOR tacitly endorsed the communist regime, trying to navigate a relationship of compromise with the atheistic authorities (Leuştean 2009). Second, the Orthodoxy's anti-abortion discourse painfully resonates in Romanians' traumatized memory with Ceauşescu's pronatalist policies (Stan and Turcescu 2005, 2007). The church waited for almost two decades after the fall of the communist regime before releasing, in 2005, an official pronouncement on abortion that defines it as the sin of infanticide in any phase. "In an effort to bridge the gap between the view of the church and the positions of the scientists and legal experts" (Stan and Turcescu 2005, 301), BOR appointed a National Commission on Bioethics that includes theologians, scientists, sociologists, and law experts. The abortion pronouncement, issued by the BOR's Committee on Bioethics, does not mention traditional contraceptive methods, like the Ogino calendar, endorsed by the Roman Catholic Church. BOR condemns the use of modern contraception as "as a very serious sin, equal to abortion." See the official website of the Romanian Patriarchat, http://patriarhia.ro/avortul-78.html; see also Stan and Turcescu (2005, 2007). However, the statement "is not a blind condemnation of abortion [and] recog-

nizes instances when abortion may be acceptable" (Stan and Turcescu 2007, 186). The impact of the pronouncement was insignificant because "with respect to abortion . . . Romanian society is far more permissive than either the church or the state" (Stan and Turcescu 2007, 197). BOR has a certain impact on maintaining a patriarchal vision of gender, as reflected in the Orthodox ritual. During the nuptial service, the priest reads St. Paul's Letter to Ephesians (5:33): "Nevertheless let every one of you in particular so love his wife even as himself; and the wife [see] that she reveres [her] husband." In what seems akin to a master and servant relation, the husband is expected to love and protect his wife, and she is asked to respect him. Another statement from the nuptial service associates the husband with the head (of the household) and the wife with the body (Miroiu 2002). These patriarchal views encoded in the Orthodox ritual may perpetuate traditional gender roles, also shaping ideas about women's reproductive health and well-being.

2. In addition to my questions about conception, other topics, such as infertility, also prompted women to mention God's will in conception. Tereza, introduced in chapter 1 as one of the women who fought infertility, told me: "I don't think that God is responsible for infertility. Usually, God *gives* children. But, you know, sometimes he gives them to the wrong people."

3. Forty-six percent (n = 20), out of forty-three interviews.

4. Delcel women's stories resonate, in both number estimates and emotional intensity, with similar abortion recollections from women quoted in other studies (Băban 1999; Kligman 1998). In this chapter, I am not as concerned with the exact number of abortions women had as I am with the practice of using abortion as a method of birth control and the role of lived religion as a reproductive decision-making resource.

5. Romania's urban-to-rural ratio is about 54 percent to 46 percent (INSSE 2011).

6. I am grateful to Sabina Stan for helping me formulate this idea.

7. Metropolitan bishop Laurențiu's anti-HPV vaccination reaction (mentioned in interlude, part 1) never became BOR's official position. Officially, BOR endorsed pediatric immunizations but not specifically the HPV vaccine. However, extremist Orthodox groups campaigned against vaccination in general and strongly opposed the HPV vaccine in particular.

4   DISMANTLING MEDICINE

1. CNAS is funded with income taxes collected through the Ministry of Finance.

2. In 2006, the Romanian parliament adopted a new health care law aimed at privatizing medical insurance, decentralizing hospital management, and regulating malpractice. The law also created a coherent legislative framework for developing national preventive and educational health programs.

3. An interactive map showed that in 2014, there were more than 500 communities (both rural and urban) with a deficit of doctors; see Alina Neagu, "Doctors Say 'Family Medicine Is Collapsing,'" *Hotnews.ro*, February 5, 2019, https://www.hotnews.ro/stiri-sanatate-22954114 -harta-interactiva-500-localitati-din-romania-medici-familie-mai-putini-decat-trebui-sau -deloc-doctorii-sustin-medicina-familie-este-colaps.htm.

4. See "Organigrama Spitalului Municipal Caritas Roșiori de Vede," n.d., http://www .spitalulcaritasrosiori.ro/images/organigrama.pdf. Another organizational chart is available at http://www.spitalulcaritasrosiori.ro/images/personal%20medical.htm.

5. In 2007, the French *Ordre National des Médecins* reported that "the number of Romanian doctors registered that year had jumped 321%" (Allen 2009, 159). A 2011 national protest organized by the medical workers' union called for the ultimate form of protest—the "strike through migration" (*greva prin emigrație*); see Dr. Florin Chirculescu, "Emigration Strike," *CriticAtac*, October 4, 2011, http://www.criticatac.ro/greva-prin-emigratie/.

6. *Antena* 3, February 8, 2009. Reforming state medicine was further complicated by political and administrative instability at the highest levels of the Health Ministry. Over three decades (1990–2020), the ministry was managed by no less than thirty-two ministers.

7. While access to specialized care within the public system is indeed contingent on a family doctor referral, patients retain, at least in theory, the right to choose their specialist.

8. In 2010, Ramona's monthly payment was the equivalent of approximately $200.

9. At the time of that conversation, I wrongly believed that vaccination was beneficial only if given before the start of the sexual life. As Alessandra Bazzano pointed out while reviewing an early draft of this chapter, the vaccine may be beneficial to sexually active individuals as well.

10. An executive order issued by Texas governor Rick Perry in February 2007 mandated "the age appropriate vaccination of all female children for HPV prior to admission to the sixth grade." The campaign produced parental anxieties, given the lack of information about the vaccine's long-term side effects. Some parents were concerned about their daughters taking advantage of the protection offered by the vaccine to engage more freely in sexually promiscuous behavior. Public health experts and doctors expressed divided opinions. The supporters of the vaccine considered its potential "to reduce the burden of cervical cancer." The critics emphasized that, since cervical cancer was not communicable, HPV was neither an urgent nor a public health threat. Suspicions of corruption rose when officials from the governor's entourage were shown to have received financial benefits from Merck (Blumenthal 2007). In India, an HPV vaccination campaign initiated in a public-private partnership and led by several nongovernmental organizations had to be canceled because of people's reluctance to allow medical practitioners the access to young girls in rural areas. The medico-scientific narratives of the vaccines as the "best" therapeutics against cervical cancer were challenged by the intended recipients. Additionally, rumors about high-level corruption made people even more reluctant to accept the vaccination for their daughters. Overall, the Indian HPV vaccination campaign was perceived as a mere substitute for a failed public health system (Towghi 2010, 2013).

5 THE OTHER HOSPITAL

1. My conversation with Doctor MT took place in 2009. At that moment, the functioning of neonatal intensive care units (NICUs) was regulated by law 95/2006. A series of executive orders from 2015, 2016, and 2017 listed all the state-financed NICUs. As of 2018, in the whole country, only one private maternity clinic (*Regina Maria* in Bucharest) was equipped for neonatal intensive care (for newborns as premature as twenty-four weeks). By 2021, a few more private hospitals have added NICU sections.

2. Informed consent was introduced in 2003. Law 95/2006 stipulates that patients eighteen years and older sign a consent form. Patients have the right to be informed of the risks associated with clinical investigations and treatments (Simionescu and Marin 2017). Personally, I was never asked to sign or to verbally provide any informed consent.

3. Like many of her peers, years after the monetary reform of 2005, Paula still refers to money using the old currency.

4. For instance, Gynia, a private maternity hospital in Cluj, offers, among others, the following ambulatory services (I converted the fees in the equivalent U.S. currency): Pap smear $65, HPV test $80, oncologic exam $47, transvaginal sonogram $35, colposcopy and biopsy $110. A vaginal birth with peridural is $1,780, while an elective C-section is $2,280 (Gynia, "Services and Rates," https://www.gynia.ro/servicii-si-tarife-ambulator/, last accessed May 17, 2021). In Romania, a middle-income country, these fees are still prohibitive to many citizens.

5. For 2020, only nine private medical practices in Roşiorii de Vede (including one obstetrical-gynecological) had a contract with the local Health Insurance House (CAS Teleorman).

6. In Romanian, in original, she said *cocograf*, an incorrect form for *ecograf*, which means ultrasound machine.

7. The main state maternity hospital in Cluj-Napoca has currently thirteen men and six women OB-GYN specialists. Out of them, four male doctors and one female doctor also hold university positions at the University of Medicine and Pharmacy. In a study carried by Ionescu and colleagues (2019), out of the seventy-three OB-GYNs interviewed, forty-three were women (58.9 percent) and thirty were men (41.1 percent).

8. In August 2018, the Health Ministry acquired eight mobile clinics for cervical cancer screenings set to start in 2019; see press release, August 22, 2018, http://www.ms.ro/2018/08 /22/ministerul-sanatatii-a-achizitionat-8-unitati-mobile-care-vor-fi-utilizate-in-programul -de-screening-pentru-cancerul-de-col-uterin/. In September 2019, the project was not yet implemented. As of May 2021, no further information was available on the Health Ministry website. See Ministry of Health, "Launch Conference of the European Public Health Challenges Program," press release, September 13, 2019, http://www.ms.ro/2019/09/13/conferinta -de-lansare-a-programului-provocari-in-sanatatea-publica-la-nivel-european/, last accessed May 17, 2021.

9. Renaşterea Foundation, https://fundatiarenasterea.ro/unitatea-mobila-de-diagnostic/, last accessed May 17, 2021.

6   LOCATING CORRUPTION

*ProTV, "Explozie la maternitatea Giuleşti din capitală!" August 18, 2010, http://stirileprotv .ro/stiri/eveniment/explozie-la-maternitatea-giulesti-din-capitala.html.

1. Corruption is embedded in "ordinary forms of sociability" that cover anything from string-pulling to a reliance on petty favors or nepotism, unwarranted fees for service, and systemic misappropriation or abuse of public goods and commission for illicit service (Blundo and Olivier de Sardan 2006, 8–9 and 81).

2. Data presented in this section was compiled from 535 articles published between January 1998 and March 2012 in three major national newspapers—*Ziua, Cotidianul,* and *Evenimentul Zilei;* from television shows from Pro TV, Antena 3, Realitatea TV, and TVR; and from articles published online on Voxpublica.ro, Contributors.ro, CriticAtac.ro, and Hotnews.ro.

3. As Romania was about to join the EU on January 1, 2007, the sanitary regulations had been revised to align Romanian hospitals to the "European standards."

4. Nineteen out of the forty-three women who talked to me in Delcel (45 percent) were unaware of their medical insurance benefits. Surveys conducted for the Romanian Center for Health Policies and Services in 2001 and 2002 show that 70 percent of rural residents had little knowledge about their rights as insured persons and made informal payments to medical staff (https://www.cpss.ro/ro/proiecte/proiecte-finalizate/156-2002.html; see also Vlădescu et al. 2008; MMT 2002). In 2005, the World Bank financed a project of "technical assistance for developing a plan to improve transparency and to decrease informal fees in the Romanian medical system." According to the World Bank study, 42 percent of people from rural and urban areas admitted to having bribed physicians and 55 percent of them said they had bribed nurses. A 2010 opinion poll shows that "85% believe that they will not get adequate care in hospital if they do not make informal payments to medical staff" (Holt 2010). Similar findings were reported more recently by Horodnic, Mazilu, and Oprea (2018).

5. In January 2009, a hidden-camera video was featured on Hotnews.ro. The video, taken by a father, showed his newborn being given a first bath by a nurse in the maternity hospital. The parent caught himself on camera slipping a paper bill into the nurse's pocket. She did not acknowledge the gesture (http://www.hotnews.ro/stiri-esential-5361458-video-spaga-maternitate -cititor-filmat-mituirea-unei-asistente.htm).

6. *Codul de deontologie medicală al colegiului medicior din Romania din 04.11.2016*, Monitorul Oficial al României (981), December 7, 2016.

7. Eugene Raikhel provided valuable suggestions about how to interpret this narrative.

8. In the European Union, food additives are given codes, composed by the letter E followed by a number.

9. Kulakov et al. (1993) reported decreased fertility rates, more birth and postpartum complications, as well as higher perinatal mortality and neonatal morbidity in affected areas from Russia, Belarus, and Ukraine. A 2006 World Health Organization (WHO) report found "no effects on fertility, numbers of stillbirths, adverse pregnancy outcomes or delivery complications" (http://www.who.int/ionizing_radiation/chernobyl/backgrounder/en/index.html). A series of studies carried by Scherb and Voigt (2009, 2012) suggests that Chernobyl ionizing radiation has contributed to an increase of congenital malformations, stillbirths, and infant deaths across Europe. Cwikel et al. (2020) found decreased fertility in women who were exposed to the radiation as young girls.

CONCLUSION

1. I draw on Gupta's conceptualization of the "discourse of corruption" as an "arena through which the state, citizens, and other organizations and aggregations come to be imagined" (1995, 376).

2. Allison Truitt helped me formulate this idea.

REFERENCES

Alexievich, Svetlana. 2016. *Secondhand Time: The Last of the Soviets*. New York: Random House.

Al-Khatib, Jamal, Christopher Robertson, and Dana-Nicoleta Lascu. 2004. "Post-Communist Consumer Ethics: The Case of Romania." *Journal of Business Ethics* 54 (1): 81–95.

Allen, Ira. 2009. "Doctors Crossing Borders: Europe's New Reality." *Canadian Medical Association Journal* 180 (2): 158–161.

American Cancer Society. 2020. "Prevent 6 Cancers with the HPV Vaccine." https://www.cancer.org/healthy/hpv-vaccine.html.

Andaya, Elise. 2009. "The Gift of Health: Socialist Medical Practice and Shifting Material and Moral Economies in Post-Soviet Cuba." *Medical Anthropology Quarterly* 23 (4): 357–374.

———. 2014. *Conceiving Cuba: Reproduction, Women, and the State in the Post-Soviet Era*. New Brunswick, NJ: Rutgers University Press.

Andreassen, Trude, Elisabete Weiderpass, Florian Nicula, Ofelia Suteu, Andreea Itu, Minodora Bumbu, Aida Tincu, Giske Ursin, and Kåre Moen. 2017. "Controversies about Cervical Cancer Screening: A Qualitative Study of Roma Women's (Non)Participation in Cervical Cancer Screening in Romania." *Social Science & Medicine* 183:48–55.

Andrei, Gabi, Lucia Efrim, and Elvira Gheorghiță. 2011. "Un an de la incendiul din Maternitatea Giulești." *Mediafax.ro*, August 16. https://www.mediafax.ro/social/un-an-de-la-incendiul-din-maternitatea-giulesti-medic-tragedia-din-2010-nu-s-ar-mai-putea-repeta-8625264.

Anton, Lorena. 2009. "On Memory Work in Post-Communist Europe: A Case Study on Romania's Ways of Remembering Its Pronatalist Past." *Anthropological Journal of European Cultures* 18 (2): 106–122.

———. 2014. "'We Will Never Speak of It Again . . .' Analyzing the Memory of Abortion in Communist Romania." *Ethnologie française* 44 (3): 421–428.

Apostol, Iuliana, Adriana Băban, Florian Nicula, Ofelia Şuteu, Daniela Coza, Camilla Amati, and Paolo Baili. 2010. "Cervical Cancer Assessment in Romania under EUROCHIP-2." *Tumori* 96:545–552.

Arbyn, Marc, Jerome Antoine, Zdravka Valerianova, Margit Magi, Aivars Stengrevics, Giedre Smailyte, Ofelia Suteu, and Andrea Micheli. 2010. "Trends in Cervical Cancer Incidence and Mortality in Bulgaria, Estonia, Latvia, Lithuania, and Romania." *Tumori* 96:517–523.

Armin, Julie. 2015. "Managing Borders, Bodies, and Cancer: Documents and the Creation of Subjects." In *Anthropologies of Cancer in Transnational Worlds*, edited by Holly F. Mathews, Nancy J. Burke, and Eirini Kampriani, 86–103. New York: Routledge.

———. 2019. "Bringing the People into Policy: Managing Cancer among Structurally Vulnerable Women." In *Negotiating Structural Vulnerability in Cancer Control*, edited by Julie Armin, Nancy J. Burke, and Laura Eichelberg, 47–68. Albuquerque: University of New Mexico Press.

Armin, Julie, Nancy J. Burke, and Laura Eichelberg, eds. 2019. *Negotiating Structural Vulnerability in Cancer Control*. Albuquerque: University of New Mexico Press.

Aronowitz, Robert. 2010. "Gardasil: A Vaccine against Cancer and a Drug to Reduce Risk." In *Three Shots at Prevention: The HPV Vaccine and the Politics of Medicine's Simple Solutions*, edited by Keith Wailoo, Julie Livingston, Steven Epstein, and Robert Aronowitz, 21–38. Baltimore: Johns Hopkins University Press.

Augé, Marc. 2009. *Non-Places: An Introduction to Supermodernity*. 2nd ed. New York: Verso.

Băban, Adriana. 1999. "From Abortion to Contraception: Romanian Experience." In *From Abortion to Contraception: A Resource to Public Policies and Reproductive Behavior in Central and Eastern Europe from 1917 to the Present*, edited by Henry P. David, 191–222. Westport, CT: Greenwood.

Băban, Adriana. 2000. "Women's Sexuality and Reproductive Behavior in post-Ceaușescu Romania: A Psychological Approach" In *Reproducing Gender: Politics, Publics and Everyday Life after Socialism*, edited by Susan Gal and Gail Kligman, 225–255. Princeton, NJ: Princeton University Press.

Băban, Adriana, Róbert Balázsi, Janet Bradley, Camelia Rusu, Aurora Szentágotai, and Raluca Tătaru. 2005. "Psychosocial and Health System Dimensions of Cervical Screening in Romania." Report by Romanian Association of Health Psychology and Engender-Health, 1–72.

Backman, Gunilla, Paul Hunt, Rajat Khosla, Camila Jaramillo-Strouss, Belachew Mekuria Fikre, Caroline Rumble, David Pevalin, David Acurio Páez, Mónica Armijos Pineda, Ariel Frisancho, Duniska Tarco, Mitra Motlagh, Dana Farcasanu, and Cristian Vladescu. 2008. "Health Systems and the Right to Health: An Assessment of 194 Countries." *Lancet* 372:2047–2085.

Balabanova, Dina, and Martin McKee. 2002. "Understanding Informal Payments for Health Care: The Example of Bulgaria." *Health Policy* 62 (3): 243–273.

Bara, Ana Claudia, W.J.A. van den Heuvel, J.A.M. Maarse, Jitse van Dijk, and Luc de Witte. 2002. "Opinions on Changes in the Romanian Health Care System from People's Point of View: A Descriptive Study." *Health Policy* 66 (2): 123–134.

Bărăscu, Magda, and Ramona Florea. 2008. "Ce ar trebui să știe mama unei fetițe de 10 ani despre vaccin?" *Hotnews.ro*, November 21. http://www.hotnews.ro/stiri-5158789-.htm?nomobile.

Bărbulescu, Elena. 1998. "Femeia și avortul în perioada 1966–1989." *Anuarul de istorie orală* 1:180–181.

Bartolini, R. M., J. L. Winkler, M. E. Penny, and D. S. LaMontagne. 2012. "Parental Acceptance of HPV Vaccine in Peru: A Decision Framework." *PloS ONE* 7 (10).

Bazylevych, Marina. 2011. "Vaccination Campaigns in Post-Socialist Ukraine: Health Care Providers Navigating Uncertainty." *Medical Anthropology Quarterly* 25 (4): 436–456.

Benard, Vicki B., Meg Watson, Mona Saraiya, Rhea Harewood, Julie S. Townsend, Antoinette M. Stroup, Hannah K. Weir, and Claudia Allemani. 2017. "Cervical Cancer Survival in the United States by Race and Stage (2001–2009): Findings from the CONCORD-2 Study." *Cancer* 123 (S24): 5119–5137.

Bennett, Elizabeth S. 1999. "Soft Truth: Ethics and Cancer in Northeast Thailand." *Anthropology & Medicine* 6 (3): 395–404.

Bennett, John W. 1998. "Classic Anthropology." *American Anthropologist* 100 (4): 951–956.

Berlinger, Nancy, and Alison Jost. 2010. "Nonmedical Exemptions to Mandatory Vaccination: Personal Belief, Public Policy, and the Ethics of Refusal." In *Three Shots at Prevention: The HPV Vaccine and the Politics of Medicine's Simple Solutions*, edited by Keith Wailoo, Julie Livingston, Steven Epstein, and Robert Aronowitz, 196–212. Baltimore: Johns Hopkins University Press.

Bernau, Anke. 2007. *Virgins: A Cultural History*. London: Granta Books.

Besnier, Niko. 2009. *Gossip and the Everyday Production of Politics*. Honolulu: University of Hawaii Press.

Betrán, A. P., J. Ye, A. B. Moller, J. Zhang, A. M. Gülmezoglu, and M. R. Torloni. 2016. "The Increasing Trend in Caesarean Section Rates: Global, Regional and National Estimates: 1990–2014." *PLoS ONE* 11 (2): e0148343.

Biehl, Joao, and Adriana Petryna, eds. 2013. *When People Come First: Critical Studies in Global Health*. Princeton, NJ: Princeton University Press.

Bizo, Aurelian, Adrian Opre, and Alina Rusu. 2014. "The Mediation Effect of Response Expectancies between Religious Coping and Non-Volitional Responses in Patients with Breast Cancer." *Journal for the Study of Religions and Ideologies* 13 (39): 181–202.

Block, Ellen, and Will McGrath. 2019. *Infected Kin: Orphan Care and AIDS in Lesotho*. New Brunswick, NJ: Rutgers University Press.

Blumenthal, Ralph. 2007. "Texas Is the First to Require Cancer Shots for School Girls." *New York Times*, February 3.

Blundo, Giorgio, and Jean-Pierre Olivier de Sardan (with N. Bako Arifari and M. Tidjani Alou). 2006. *Everyday Corruption and the State: Citizens and Public Officials in Africa*. Cape Town: Zed Books.

Boia, Lucian. 2016. *Strania Istorie a Comunismului Românesc (și Nefericitele Ei Consecințe)*. București: Humanitas.

Boonmongkon, Pimpawun, Jen Pylypa, and Mark Nichter. 1999. "Emerging Fears of Cervical Cancer in Northeast Thailand." *Anthropology & Medicine* 6 (3): 359–380.

Bourdieu, Pierre. 1990. *The Logic of Practice*. Translated by Richard Nice. Cambridge: Polity Press.

Bouzarovski, Stefan, Luděk Sýkora, and Roman Matoušek. 2016. "Locked-In Post-Socialism: Rolling Path Dependencies in Liberec's District Heating System." *Eurasian Geography and Economics* 57 (4–5): 624–642.

Brădățan, Cristina, and G. Firebaugh. 2007. "History, Population Policies, and Fertility Decline in Eastern Europe: A Case Study." *Journal of Family History* 32 (2): 1–14.

Bray, Freddie, Anja H. Loos, Peter McCarron, Elizabete Weiderpass, Mark Arbyn, Henrik Møller, Matti Hakama, and D. Max Parkin. 2005. "Trends in Cervical Squamous Cell Carcinoma Incidence in 13 European Countries: Changing Risk and the Effects of Screening." *Cancer Epidemiology, Biomarkers and Prevention* 14 (3): 677–686.

Brison, Susan. 1999. "Trauma Narratives and the Remaking of the Self." In *Acts of Memory: Cultural Recall in the Present*, edited by Mieke Bal, Jonathan Crewe, and Leo Spitzer, 39–54. Hanover, NH: Dartmouth College—University Press of New England.

Brotherton, Sean P. 2012. *Revolutionary Medicine: Health and the Body in Post-Soviet Cuba*. Durham, NC: Duke University Press.

Bruni, L., G. Albero, B. Serrano, M. Mena, D. Gómez, J. Muñoz, F. X. Bosch, and S. de Sanjosé. 2019. "Human Papillomavirus and Related Diseases in Romania." Summary Report. Catalan Institute of Oncology and the International Agency for Research on Cancer (ICO/IARC), Information Centre on HPV and Cancer (HPV Information Centre).

Buchel, Christoph, and Giovanni Carmine. 2008. *Ceau*. Göttingen: Steidl; London: Thames & Hudson.

Butler, Judith. 1997. *The Psychic Life of Power: Theories in Subjection*. Palo Alto, CA: Stanford University Press.

Campion-Vincent, Véronique, and Nancy Scheper-Hughes. 2001. "On Organ Theft Narratives." *Current Anthropology* 42 (4): 555–558.

Cărtărescu, Mircea. 2010. "Uciderea pruncilor." *Evenimentul Zilei*, August 20. http://www.evz.ro/detalii/stiri/senatul-evz-uciderea-pruncilor-903620.html.

CDC. 2021. "What Should I Know about Screening?" Centers for Disease Control and Prevention. https://www.cdc.gov/cancer/cervical/basic_info/screening.htm.

Chapman, Rachel. 2010. *Family Secrets: Risking Reproduction in Central Mozambique*. Nashville: Vanderbilt University Press.

Chavez, L. R., F. A. Hubbell, J. M. McMullin, R. G. Martinez, and S. I. Mishra. 1995. "Structure and Meaning in Models of Breast and Cervical Cancer Risk Factors: A Comparison of Perceptions among Latinas, Anglo Women, and Physicians." *Medical Anthropology Quarterly* 9 (1): 40–74.

Chavez, Leo R., Juliet M. McMullin, Shiraz I. Mishra, and Allan Hubbell. 2001. "Beliefs Matter: Cultural Beliefs and the Use of Cervical Cancer-Screening Tests." *American Anthropologist* 103 (4): 1114–1129.

Chenhall, R. D., and K. Senior. 2018. "Living the Social Determinants of Health: Assemblages in a Remote Aboriginal Community." *Medical Anthropology Quarterly* 32 (2): 177–195.

Chirculescu, Florin. 2011. "Sănătatea este un drept. Nu se poate privatiza totul. Tuberculoza nu e privatizabilă." *CriticAtac*, October 6. http://www.criticatac.ro/10402/sanatatea-este-un-drept-nu-se-poate-privatiza-totul-tuberculoza-nu-e-privatizabila/.

Clifford, James, and George Marcus. 1986. *Writing Culture: The Poetics and Politics of Ethnography*. Berkeley: University of California Press.

Coleman, Maame Aba, Judy Levison, and Haleh Sangi-Haghpeykar. 2011. "HPV Vaccine Acceptability in Ghana, West Africa." *Vaccine* 29 (23): 3945–3950.

Colen, Shellee. 1995. "'Like a Mother to Them': Stratified Reproduction and West Indian Childcare Workers and Employers in New York." In *Conceiving the New World Order: The Global Politics of Reproduction*, edited by Faye D. Ginsburg and Rayna Rapp, 78–102. Berkeley: University of California Press.

Connell, Erin, and Alan Hunt. 2010. "The HPV Vaccination Campaign: A Project of Moral Regulation in an Era of Biopolitics." *Canadian Journal of Sociology* 35 (1): 63–82.

Crăciun, Catrinel, and Adriana Băban. 2012. "Who Will Take the Blame? Understanding the Reasons Why Romanian Mothers Decline HPV Vaccination for their Daughters." *Vaccine* 30 (48): 6789–6793.

Crăciun, Catrinel, Irina Todorova, and Adriana Băban. 2018. "Taking Responsibility for My Health: Health System Barriers and Women's Attitudes toward Cervical Cancer Screening in Romania and Bulgaria." *Journal of Health Psychology* 25 (13–14): 2151–2163.

Creangă, Ion. (1875) 1978. *Memories of My Boyhood: Stories and Tales*. Translated from Romanian by Ana Cartianu. Bucharest: Minerva.

Cucu, Maria Alexandra. 2020. *Raport Național Privind Starea de Sănătate a Populației României 2019*. București: Institutul Național de Statistică.

Cwikel, J., R. Sergienko, G. Gutvirtz, R. Abramovitz, D. Slusky, M. Quastel, and E. Sheiner. 2020. "Reproductive Effects of Exposure to Low-Dose Ionizing Radiation: A Long-Term Follow-Up of Immigrant Women Exposed to the Chernobyl Accident." *Journal of Clinical Medicine* 9 (6): 1786.

Daley, E. M., C. A. Vamos, E. L. Thompson, G. D. Zimet, Z. Rosberger, L. Merrell, and N. S. Kline. 2017. "The Feminization of HPV: How Science, Politics, Economics and Gender Norms Shaped U.S. HPV Vaccine Implementation." *Papillomavirus Research* 3:142–148.

David, Henry, and Adriana Băban. 1996. "Women's Health and Reproductive Rights: Romanian Experience." *Patient Education and Counseling* 28:235–245.

David, Henry P. 1999. "Overview." In *From Abortion to Contraception: A Resource to Public Policies and Reproductive Behavior in Central and Eastern Europe from 1917 to the Present*, edited by Henry P. David, 3–22. Westport, CT: Greenwood.

David, Ioana. 2010. "Maternitățile private pun presiune pe sistemul de stat: una din zece femei alege să nască la privat în capital." *Ziarul Financiar*, October 7. http://www.zf.ro/companii

/maternitatile-private-pun-presiune-pe-sistemul-de-stat-una-din-zece-femei-alege-sa
-nasca-la-privat-in-capitala-7455471/.

Davis-Floyd, Robbie. 2003. *Birth as an American Rite of Passage.* 2nd ed. Berkeley: University of California Press.

De Certeau, Michel. (1984) 2011. *The Practice of Everyday Life.* Berkeley: University of California Press.

———. 2005. "The Practice of Everyday Life: Making Do: Uses and Tactics." In *Practicing History: New Directions in Historical Writing after the Linguistic Turn,* edited by Gabrielle M. Speigel, 217–227. New York: Routledge.

Derrida, Jacques. (1994) 2006. *Specters of Marx: The State of the Debt, the Work of Mourning and the New International.* New York: Routledge.

De Sanjosé, Silvia, Mireia Diaz, Xavier Castellsagué, Gary Clifford, Laia Bruni, Nubia Muñoz, and Xavier Bosch. 2007. "Worldwide Prevalence and Genotype Distribution of Cervical Human Papillomavirus DNA in Women with Normal Cytology: A Meta-Analysis." *Lancet Infectious Disease* 7:453–459.

DEX. 1998. *Dicționarul Explicativ al Limbii Române.* Bucharest: Univers Enciclopedic.

Dilger, H., S. Huschke, and D. Mattes. 2015. "Ethics, Epistemology, and Engagement: Encountering Values in Medical Anthropology." *Medical Anthropology* 34 (1): 1–10.

Doboș, Corina, Luciana Jinga, and Florin Soare. 2010. *Politica pronatalistă a regimului Ceaușescu: o perspectivă comparativă.* Iași: Polirom.

Dobreanu, Cristina, Ondine Ghergut, and Andreea Pocotilă. 2010. "Tragedia din maternitate. Aparatul de aer condiționat nu era pentru spital." *România Liberă,* August 18. https://romanialibera.ro/special/tragedia-din-maternitate-aparatul-de-aer-conditionat-nu-era-pentru-spital-196894.

Dobrescu, Petre. 2010. "Coșmarul mamelor de la Maternitatea Giulești: 'Doamne, nu-mi lua pruncul!'" *Libertatea.ro,* August 17. http://www.libertatea.ro/detalii/articol/cosmarul-mamelor-de-la-maternitatea-giulesti-doamne-nu-mi-lua-pruncul-300104.html.

Domnișoru, Ciprian. 2011. "Reforma Băsescu în Sănătate: segmentarea consumatorilor." *CriticAtac,* September 27. https://www.criticatac.ro/reforma-basescu-in-sanatate-segmentarea-consumatorilor/.

Douglas, Mary. 1969. *Purity and Danger: An Analysis of Concepts of Pollution and Taboo.* London: Routledge & Kegan Paul.

Dudgeon, M. R., and M. C. Inhorn. 2004. "Men's Influences on Women's Reproductive Health: Medical Anthropological Perspectives." *Social Science & Medicine* 59 (7): 1379–1395.

Du Plessix Gray, Francine. 1989. *Soviet Women Walking the Tightrope.* New York: Doubleday.

Durandin, Catherine, and Zoe Petre. 2010. *Romania since 1989.* Boulder, CO: East European Monographs; New York: Columbia University Press.

Einarsdóttir, Jónína. 2000. *"Tired of Weeping": Child Death and Mourning among Papel Mothers in Guinea-Bissau.* Stockholm: Dept. of Social Anthropology, Stockholm University.

Eliot, T. S. (1921) 1997. *The Sacred Wood and Early Major Essays.* Mineola, NY: Dover Publications.

Elman, Colin, John Gerring, and James Mahoney. 2016. "Case Study Research: Putting the Quant into the Qual." *Sociological Methods & Research* 45 (3): 375–391.

Erdman, Joanna N. 2014. "Procedural Abortion Rights: Ireland and the European Court of Human Rights." *Reproductive Health Matters* 22 (44): 22–30.

Evans-Pritchard, Edward. (1937) 1976. *Witchcraft, Oracles and Magic among the Azande.* Abr. ed. Oxford: Oxford University Press.

Fărcăşanu, Dana Otilia. 2010. "Population Perception on Corruption, Informal Payments and Introduction of Co-payments in the Public Health System in Romania." *Management in Health* XIV (1): 8.

Farmer, Paul. 2001. *Infections and Inequalities: The Modern Plagues.* Berkeley: University of California Press.

Fassin, Didier. 2007. *When Bodies Remember: Experiences and Politics of AIDS in South Africa.* Berkeley: University of California Press.

Feldman-Savelsberg, Pamela, Flavien Ndonko, and Bergis Schmidt-Ehry. 2000. "Sterilizing Vaccines or the Politics of the Womb: Retrospective Study of a Rumor in Cameroon." *Medical Anthropology Quarterly* 14 (2): 159–179.

Ferris, D. G., J. Shapiro, C. Fowler, C. Cutler, J. Waller, and W. S. Guevara Condorhuaman. 2015. "The Impact of Accessible Cervical Cancer Screening in Perú–The Día del Mercado Project." *Journal of Lower Genital Tract Disease* 19 (3): 229–233.

Ferzacca, Steve. 2000. "'Actually, I Don't Feel That Bad': Managing Diabetes and the Clinical Encounter." *Medical Anthropology Quarterly* 14 (1): 28–50.

Florea Marian, Simion. (1892) 2009. *Naşterea la români.* Bucureşti: Seculum.

Flórez, Karen, Alejandra Aguirre, Anahí Viladrich, Amarilis Céspedes, Ana Alicia De La Cruz, and Ana Abraído-lanza. 2009. "Fatalism or Destiny? A Qualitative Study and Interpretative Framework on Dominican Women's Breast Cancer Beliefs." *Journal of Immigrant and Minority Health* 11 (4): 291–301.

Fordyce, Lauren, and Aminata Maraesa, eds. 2012. *Risk, Reproduction, and Narratives of Experience.* Nashville: Vanderbilt University Press.

Foucault, Michel. 1977. *Discipline and Punish: The Birth of the Prison.* New York: Vintage Books.

———. 1982. "The Subject and Power." *Critical Inquiry* 8 (4): 777–795.

———. 1994 (1963). *The Birth of the Clinic: An Archaeology of Medical Perception.* New York: Vintage Books.

Franklin, Sarah, and Helena Ragoné. 1998. *Reproducing Reproduction: Kinship, Power, and Technological Innovation.* Philadelphia: University of Pennsylvania Press.

Friedman, Jack. 2009. "The 'Social Case': Illness, Psychiatry, and Deinstitutionalization in Postsocialist Romania." *Medical Anthropology Quarterly* 23 (4): 375–396.

Fumurescu, Alin. 2011. ". . . România avortată." *Cuvântul Ortodox,* February 22. http://www.cuvantul-ortodox.ro/recomandari/articolele-saptamanii-1-cum-s-a-avortat-romania-singura-e-o-intreaga-lume-pe-care-am-avortat-o-o-intreaga-istorie-care-ar-fi-aratat-cu-totul-altfel/.

Gal, Peter, and Martin McKee. 2005. "Fee-for-Service or Donation? Hungarian Perspectives on Informal Payment for Health Care." *Social Science & Medicine* 60:1445–1457.

Gal, Susan, and Gail Kligman. 2000. *The Politics of Gender after Socialism.* Princeton, NJ: Princeton University Press.

Garland, David. 2014. "What Is a "History of the Present"? On Foucault's Genealogies and Their Critical Preconditions." *Punishment & Society* 16 (4): 365–384.

Gheorghe, Dan. 2011. "Cum a ajuns România să aibă 22 de milioane de avorturi?" *România Liberă,* February 20. https://romanialibera.ro/special/reportaje/cum-a-ajuns-romania-sa-aiba-22-milioane-de-avorturi-217321.

Ghodsee, Kristen. 2011. *Lost in Transition: Ethnographies of Everyday Life after Communism.* Durham, NC: Duke University Press.

Ginsburg, Faye, and Rayna Rapp. 1995. *Conceiving the New World Order: The Global Politics of Reproduction.* Berkeley: University of California Press.

Ginsburg, O., F. Bray, M. P. Coleman, V. Vanderpuye, A. Eniu, S. R. Kotha, M. Sarker, T. T. Huong, C. Allemani, A. Dvaladze, J. Gralow, K. Yeates, C. Taylor, N. Oomman, S. Krishnan, R. Sullivan, D. Kombe, M. M. Blas, G. Parham, N. Kassami, and L. Conteh. 2017. "The Global Burden of Women's Cancers: A Grand Challenge in Global Health." *Lancet* 389 (10071): 847–860.

Good, Byron. 1994. *Medicine, Rationality and Experience: An Anthropological Perspective*. Cambridge: Cambridge University Press.

———. 2020. "Hauntology: Theorizing the Spectral in Psychological Anthropology." *Ethos* 47 (4): 411–426.

Gottlieb, Alma. 2004. *The Afterlife Is Where We Come From: The Culture of Infancy in West Africa*. Chicago: University of Chicago Press.

Gottlieb, Samantha D. 2018. *Not Quite a Cancer Vaccine: Selling HPV and Cervical Cancer*. New Brunswick, NJ: Rutgers University Press.

Gregg, Jessica. 2003. *Virtually Virgins: Sexual Strategies and Cervical Cancer in Recife, Brazil*. Palo Alto, CA: Stanford University Press.

———. 2011. "An Unanticipated Source of Hope: Stigma and Cervical Cancer in Brazil." *Medical Anthropology Quarterly* 25 (1): 70–84.

Grielen, Saskia, Wienke Boerma, and Peter Groenewegen. 2000. "Unity or Diversity? Task Profiles of General Practitioners in Central and Eastern Europe." *European Journal of Public Health* 10:249–254.

Grigore, Mihaela, Răzvan Popovici, Anda Pristavu, Ana Maria Grigore, Mioara Matei, and Dumitru Gafitanu. 2017. "Perception and Use of Pap Smear Screening among Rural and Urban Women in Romania." *European Journal of Public Health* 27 (6): 1084–1088.

Grigore, Valentina. 2009. "Bebeluș ars după ce a fost uitat de asistentă în incubator." *România Liberă*, November 16. https://romanialibera.ro/special/bebelus-ars-dupa-ce-a-fost-uitat-de-asistenta-in-incubator-170060/.

Gupta, Akhil. 1995. "Blurred Boundaries: The Discourse of Corruption, the Culture of Politics, and the Imagined State." *American Ethnologist* 22 (2): 375–402.

Gupta, Akhil, and Aradhana Sharma, eds. 2006. *The Anthropology of the State: A Reader*. Malden, MA: Blackwell Publishing.

Gutmann, Matthew. 2011. "Planning Men Out of Family Planning: A Case Study." In *Reproduction, Globalization, and the State: New Theoretical and Ethnographic Perspectives*, edited by Carole H. Browner and Carolyn F. Sargent, 53–67. Durham, NC: Duke University Press.

Haas, M., T. Ashton, K. Blum, T. Christiansen, E. Conis, L. Crivelli, M. K. Lim, M. Lisac, M. MacAdam, and S. Schlette. 2009. "Drugs, Sex, Money and Power: An HPV Vaccine Case Study." *Health Policy* 92 (2–3): 288–295.

Hakama, Matti, Michel Coleman, Delia-Marina Alexe, and Anssi Auvinen. 2008. "Cancer Screening: Evidence and Practice in Europe 2008." *European Journal of Cancer* 44:1404–1413.

Hann, Chris, and Hermann Goltz, eds. 2010. *Eastern Christians in Anthropological Perspective*. Berkeley: University of California Press.

Hannerz, Ulf. 2006. "Studying Down, Up, Sideways, Through, Backwards, Forwards, Away and at Home: Reflections on the Field Worries of an Expansive Discipline." In *Locating the Field: Space, Place and Context in Anthropology*, edited by Simon Coleman and Peter Collins, 23–41. Oxford: Berg.

Hărăguș, Mihaela. 2014. "Intergenerational Solidarity in Co-Residential Living Arrangements." *Revista de Asistență Socială* 4:27–42.

Harper, Krista. 2001. "Chernobyl Stories and Anthropological Shock in Hungary." *Anthropological Quarterly* 74 (3): 114–123.

Harvey, David. 2007. *A Brief History of Neoliberalism*. Oxford: Oxford University Press.

Harvey, T. S. 2011. "Maya Mobile Medicine in Guatemala: The 'Other' Public Health." *Medical Anthropology Quarterly* 25 (1): 47–69.

Heller, Alison. 2019. *Fistula Politics: Birthing Injuries and the Quest for Continence in Niger*. New Brunswick, NJ: Rutgers University Press.

Heller, Jacob. 2008. *The Vaccine Narrative*. Nashville: Vanderbilt University Press.

Holt, Ed. 2010. "Romania's Health System Lurches into New Crisis." *Lancet* 376 (9748): 1211–1212.

Hopkins, Kristine. 2000. "Are Brazilian Women Really Choosing to Deliver by Cesarean?" *Social Science & Medicine* 51 (5): 725–740.

Horodnic, Adrian, Sorin Mazilu, and Liviu Oprea. 2018. "Drivers behind Widespread Informal Payments in the Romanian Public Health Care System: From Tolerance to Corruption to Socio-Economic and Spatial Patterns." *International Journal of Health Planning and Management* 33 (2–3).

Iepan, Florin. 2005. *The Children of the Decree*. Documentary, February 28, 2012. Video, 1:07:40. http://www.youtube.com/watch?v=ZgZJ-IV8Eto.

Ilişiu, Minodora Bianca, Dana Hashim, Trude Andreassen, Nathalie C. Støer, Florian Nicula, and Elisabete Weiderpass. 2019. "HPV Testing for Cervical Cancer in Romania: High-Risk HPV Prevalence among Ethnic Subpopulations and Regions." *Annals of Global Health* 85 (1): 89.

Inhorn, Marcia. 2006. "Defining Women's Health: A Dozen Messages from More than 150 Ethnographies." *Medical Anthropology Quarterly* 20 (3): 345–378.

———. 2012. *The New Arab Man: Emergent Masculinities, Technologies, and Islam in the Middle East*. Princeton, NJ: Princeton University Press.

INSSE. 2011. "Recensământul populației și al locuințelor." *Institutul Național de Statistică*. http://www.recensamantromania.ro/noutati/volumul-ii-populatia-stabila-rezidenta-structura-etnica-si-confesionala/.

Ionescu, Cringu Antoniu, Mihai Dimitriu, Elena Poenaru, Mihai Bănacu, Gheorghe Otto Furău, Dan Navolan, and Liana Ples. 2019. "Defensive Caesarean Section: A Reality and a Recommended Health Care Improvement for Romanian Obstetrics." *Journal of Evaluation in Clinical Practice* 25 (1): 111–116.

Ionescu, Simona. 2015. "Adevăruri spuse doar la tribunal! Ce s-a întâmplat la Maternitatea Giulești, când 11 bebeluși au fost prinși în incendiu." *Evenimentul Zilei*, April 6. https://evz.ro/adevaruri-spuse-doar-la-tribunal-ce-s-a-intamplat-la-maternitatea-giulesti-cand-11-bebelusi-au-fost-prinsi-in-incendiu.html.

Iosif, Anamaria. 2003. "Healing, Orthodoxy, and Personhood in Post-Socialist Romania." PhD thesis, Tulane University.

Irimie, Sorina, Mariana Vlad, Ileana Mireștean, Ovidiu Bălăcescu, Meda Rus, Loredana Bălăcescu, Ioana Berindan-Neagoe, Rareș Buiga, Claudia Ordeanu, Viorica Nagy, and Alexandru Irimie. 2011. "Risk Factors in a Sample of Patients with Advanced Cervical Cancer." *Applied Medical Informatics* 29:1–10.

Jain, Lochlann S. 2013. *Malignant: How Cancer Becomes Us*. Berkeley: University of California Press.

Jinga, Luciana. 2015. *Gen și reprezentare în România comunistă: 1944–1989*. Iași: Polirom.

Jinga, Luciana, Corina Doboș, Florin Soare, and Cristina Roman. 2011. *Politica pro-natalistă a regimului Ceaușescu*. Iași: Polirom.

Johnson, Brooke, Mihai Horga, and Peter Fajans. 2004. "A Strategic Assessment of Abortion and Contraception in Romania." *Reproductive Health Matters* 12 (24): 184–194.

Johnson, Kimberly. 2006. "'You Just Do Your Part. God Will Do the Rest': Spirituality and Culture in the Medical Encounter." *Southern Medical Journal* 99 (10): 1163.

Kaneff, Deema. 2002. "Why People Don't Die 'Naturally' Any More: Changing Relations between 'The Individual' and 'The State' in Post-Socialist Bulgaria." *Journal of the Royal Anthropological Institute* 8 (1): 89–105.

Kant, Immanuel. (1781) 2018. *The Critique of Pure Reason.* Translated by J.M.D. Meiklejohn. Overland Park, KS: Digireads.com Publishing.

Kapsalis, Terri. 1997. *Public Privates: Performing Gynecology from Both Ends of the Speculum.* Durham, NC: Duke University Press.

Kaufman, Sharon. 2010. "Regarding the Rise in Autism: Vaccine Safety Doubt, Conditions of Inquiry, and the Shape of Freedom." *Ethos* 38 (1): 8–32.

Keil, Thomas, and Viviana Andreescu. 1999. "Fertility Policy in Ceauşescu's Romania." *Journal of Family History* 24 (4): 478–492.

Kelly, Patricia, Molly Allison, and Megha Ramaswamy. 2018. "Cervical Cancer Screening among Incarcerated Women." *PLoS ONE* 13 (6): e0199220.

Kideckel, David. 1993. *The Solitude of Collectivism: Romanian Villagers to the Revolution and Beyond.* Ithaca, NY: Cornell University Press.

———. 2008. *Getting By in Postsocialist Romania: Labor, the Body and Working-Class Culture.* Bloomington: Indiana University Press.

Kipnis, Andrew. 1997. *Producing Guanxi: Sentiment, Self and Subculture in a North China Village.* Durham, NC: Duke University Press.

Kligman, Gail. 1988. *The Wedding of the Dead: Ritual, Poetics, and Popular Culture in Transylvania.* Berkeley: University of California Press.

———. 1995. "Political Demography: The Banning of Abortion in Ceausescu's Romania." In *Conceiving the New World Order: The Global Politics of Reproduction,* edited by Faye Ginsburg and Rayna Rapp, 234–255. Berkeley: University of California Press.

———. 1998. *The Politics of Duplicity: Controlling Reproduction in Ceausescu's Romania.* Berkeley: University of California Press.

Kohler, Hans-Peter, Francesco C. Billari, and José A. Ortega. 2006. "Low Fertility in Europe: Causes, Implications and Policy Options." In *The Baby Bust: Who Will Do the Work? Who Will Pay the Taxes?,* edited by F. R. Harris, 48–109. Lanham, MD: Rowman & Littlefield Publishers.

Konrad, Monica. 2005. *Narrating the New Predictive Genetics: Ethics, Ethnography, and Science.* Cambridge: Cambridge University Press.

Krause, Elizabeth, and Silvia DeZordo. 2012. "Introduction. Ethnography and Biopolitics: Tracing 'Rationalities' of Reproduction across the North–South Divide." *Anthropology & Medicine* 19 (2).

Kulakov, V. I., T. N. Sokur, A. I. Volobuev, I. S. Tzibulskaya, V. A. Malisheva, B. I. Zikin, L. C. Ezova, L. A. Belyaeva, P. D. Bonartzev, N. V. Speranskaya, J. M. Tchesnokova, N. K. Matveeva, E. S. Kaliznuk, L. B. Miturova, and N. S. Orlova. 1993. "Female Reproductive Function in Areas Affected by Radiation after the Chernobyl Power Station Accident." *Environmental Health Perspectives* 101:117–123.

Kutzin, Joseph, Melitta Jakab, and Cheryl Cashin. 2010. "Lessons from Health Financing Reform in Central and Eastern Europe and the Former Soviet Union." *Health Economics, Policy and Law* 5 (2):135–147.

Lakoff, George, and Mark Johnson. (1980) 2003. *Metaphors We Live By.* Chicago: University of Chicago Press.

Leach, Melissa, and James Fairhead. 2007. *Vaccine Anxieties: Global Science, Child Health and Society.* Abingdon, UK: Earthscan Routledge.

Laslo, Cecilia. 2018. "Vaccinul Care N-a Străpuns." https://www.scena9.ro/article/vaccin -hpv.

Laslo, Cecilia. 2019. "Vaccinul Care M-a Străpuns." https://www.scena9.ro/article/vaccin -hpv-romania.

Ledeneva, Alena. 2006. *How Russia Really Works: The Informal Practices That Shaped Post-Soviet Politics and Business.* Ithaca, NY: Cornell University Press.

Lende, D. H., and A. Lachiondo. 2009. "Embodiment and Breast Cancer among African American Women." *Qualitative Health Research* 19 (2): 216–228.

Leuștean, Lucian. 2009. *Orthodoxy and the Cold War: Religion and Political Power in Romania, 1947–65.* New York: Palgrave Macmillan.

Livingston, Julie. 2012. *Improvising Medicine: An African Oncology Ward in an Emerging Cancer Epidemic.* Durham, NC: Duke University Press.

Lock, Margaret. 1993. *Encounters with Aging: Mythologies of Menopause in Japan and North America.* Berkeley: University of California Press.

Lock, Margaret, and Patricia Kaufert, eds. 1998. *Pragmatic Women and Body Politics.* New York: Cambridge University Press.

Lock, Margaret, and Vihn-Kim Nguyen. 2010. *An Anthropology of Biomedicine.* New York: Wiley-Blackwell.

Lora-Wainwright, Anna. 2013. *Fighting for Breath: Living Morally and Dying of Cancer in a Chinese Village.* Honolulu: University of Hawaii Press.

Luque, J. S., and H. Castañeda. 2013. "Delivery of Mobile Clinic Services to Migrant and Seasonal Farmworkers: A Review of Practice Models for Community-Academic Partnerships." *Journal of Community Health* 38:397–407.

Magyari-Vincze, Eniko. 2006. "Romanian Gender Regimes and Women's Citizenship." In *Women and Citizenship in Central and Eastern Europe,* edited by Jasmina Lukić, Joanna Regulska and Daria Zaviršek, 21–37. Farnham, UK: Ashgate Publishing.

Manderson, Lenore. 1999. "Gender, Normality and the Post-Surgical Body." *Anthropology & Medicine* 6 (3): 381–394.

———. 2011. *Surface Tensions: Surgery, Bodily Boundaries and the Social Self.* Walnut Creek, CA: Left Coast Press.

———. 2015. "Cancer Enigmas and Agendas." In *Anthropologies of Cancer in Transnational Worlds,* edited by Holly F. Mathews, Nancy J. Burke, and Eirini Kampriani, 241–254. New York: Routledge.

Manderson, Lenore, and Narelle Warren. 2016. "'Just One Thing after Another': Recursive Cascades and Chronic Conditions. *Medical Anthropology Quarterly* 30 (4): 479–497.

Martinez, Rebecca. 2018. *Marked Women: The Cultural Politics of Cervical Cancer in Venezuela.* Palo Alto, CA: Stanford University Press.

Martinez, R. G., L. R. Chavez, and F. A. Hubbell. 1997. "Purity and Passion: Risk and Morality in Latina Immigrants' and Physicians' Beliefs about Cervical Cancer." *Medical Anthropology* 17 (4): 337–362.

Masquelier, Adeline. 2012. "Public Health or Public Threat? Polio Eradication Campaigns, Islamic Revival, and the Materialization of State Power in Niger." In *Medicine, Mobility and Power in Global Africa: Transnational Health and Healing,* edited by Hansjörg Dilger, Abdoulaye Kane, and Stacey A. Langwick, 213–240. Bloomington: Indiana University Press.

Mathews, Holly F., Nancy J. Burke, and Eirini Kampriani, eds. 2015. *Anthropologies of Cancer in Transnational Worlds.* New York: Routledge.

Maver, Polona J., Katja Seme, Tina Korać, Goran Dimitrov, Lajos Döbrőssy, Ludmila Engele, Ermina Iljazović, Vesna Kesić, Petya Kostova, Dragan Lauševic, Anita Maurina, Florian A Nicula, Yulia Panayotova, Maja Primic Žakelj, Alenka Repše Fokter, Ewa Romejko-Wolniewicz, Giedrė Smailytė, Ofelia Şuteu, Joanna Świderska-Kiec, Ruth Tachezy, Zdravka Valerianova, Piret Veerus, Ilze Vīberga, Ariana Znaor, Pavol Zubor, and Mario Poljak. 2013. "Cervical Cancer Screening Practices in Central and Eastern Europe in 2012." *Acta Dermatovenerologica Alpina, Pannonica, et Adriatica* 22:7–19.

McGuire, Meredith. 2008. *Lived Religion: Faith and Practice in Everyday Life*. Oxford: Oxford University Press.

McKie, Linda. 1995. "The Art of Surveillance or Reasonable Prevention? The Case of Cervical Screening." *Sociology of Health & Illness* 17 (4): 441–457.

Mcmullin, Juliet M., Israel De Alba, Leo R. Chávez, and F. Allan Hubbell. 2005. "Influence of Beliefs about Cervical Cancer Etiology on Pap Smear Use among Latina Immigrants." *Ethnicity & Health* 10 (1): 3–18.

McRee, Annie-Laurie, Paul Reiter, Sami Gottlieb, and Noel Brewer. 2011. "Mother-Daughter Communication about HPV Vaccine." *Journal of Adolescent Health* 48 (3): 314–317.

Mendes Lobão, W., F. G. Duarte, J. D. Burns, C. A. de Souza Teles Santos, M. C. Chagas de Almeida, A. Reingold, and E. Duarte Moreira Junior. 2018. "Low Coverage of HPV Vaccination in the National Immunization Programme in Brazil: Parental Vaccine Refusal or Barriers in Health-Service Based Vaccine Delivery?" *PloS ONE* 13 (11).

Metzl, Jonathan. 2019. *Dying of Whiteness: How the Politics of Racial Resentment Is Killing America's Heartland*. New York: Basic Books.

Mihăilescu, Vintilă. 2007. *Anthropologie: Cinci Introduceri*. Iaşi: Polirom.

Mihalache, Georgiana. 2019. "Dacă nu s-ar da otova banii în mediul de stat, n-ar avea timp să-şi formeze şi clinică privată." *Ziarul Financiar*. https://www.zf.ro/eveniment/ludovic-orban-premierul-romaniei-despre-medicii-care-lucreaza-in-paralel-la-stat-si-la-privat-daca-nu-s-ar-da-otova-banii-in-mediul-de-stat-n-ar-avea-timp-sa-si-formeze-si-clinica-privata-18551356.

Miroiu, Mihaela. 2002. "Fetzele Patriarhatului/ Faces of Patriarchy." *Journal for the Study of Religions and Ideologies* 1 (3): 208.

———. 2010. "'Not the Right Moment!' Women and the Politics of Endless Delay in Romania." *Women's History Review* 19 (4): 575–593.

Miroiu, Mihaela, and Otilia Dragomir, eds. 2010. *Naşterea: Istorii trăite*. Iaşi: Polirom.

Mishtal, Joanna. 2009. "Matters of 'Conscience': The Politics of Reproductive Healthcare in Poland." *Medical Anthropology Quarterly* 23 (2):161–183.

———. 2015. *The Politics of Morality: The Church, the State and Reproductive Rights in Postsocialist Poland*. Athens: Ohio University Press.

Mixich, Vlad. 2010. "Cucuvelele." *DW.com*, August 18. https://www.dw.com/ro/cucuvelele/a-5919577.

MMT. 2002. "Barometrul de opinie privind serviciile de sănătate realizat în rîndul populaţiei din România." (Public Opinion Barometer Regarding Health Care Services among Romanians). Sondaj realizat de Metro Media Transilvania la cererea Centrului pentru Politici şi Servicii de Sănătate.

Mouallif, M., H. L. Bowyer, S. Festali, A. Albert, Y. Filali-Zegzouti, S. Guenin, P. Delvenne, J. Waller, and M. M. Ennaji. 2014. "Cervical Cancer and HPV: Awareness and Vaccine Acceptability among Parents in Morocco." *Vaccine* 32 (3): 409–416.

Murthy, Padmini, and Clyde Landford Smith. 2010. *Women's Global Health and Human Rights*. Sudbury, MA: Jones and Bartlett Publishers.

Neagu, Alina. 2009. "Ministrul Sănătăţii: Doar 2,57% dintre elevele de clasa a patra au fost vaccinate împotriva cancerului de col uterin. Motivul eşecului campaniei—lipsa informării populaţiei." *Hotnews.ro*, January 18. https://m.hotnews.ro/stire/5338565?amp.

O'Neill, Bruce. 2017. *The Space of Boredom: Homelessness in the Slowing Global Order.* Durham, NC: Duke University Press.

Ong, Aihwa. 2006. *Neoliberalism as Exception: Mutations in Citizenship and Sovereignty.* Durham, NC: Duke University Press.

Ortner, Sherry B. 1995. "Resistance and the Problem of Ethnographic Refusal." *Comparative Studies in Society and History* 37 (1): 173–193.

Păduraru, Alina, and Andrei Udişteanu. 2018. "Naştem şi noi azi?" *Recorder*, February 1. https://recorder.ro/nastem-si-noi-azi-industria-cezarienelor-alimentata-de-teama-comoditate-si-lacomie-video/.

Pârvulescu, Ioana, ed. 2015. *Şi eu am trăit în comunism.* Bucureşti: Humanitas.

Paveliu, Sorin. 2011. "Despre privatizarea în sănătate ca soluţie la criza permanentă a sistemului." *CriticAtac*, September 28. http://www.criticatac.ro/10254/despre-privatizarea-in-sanatate-ca-solutie-la-criza-permanenta-a-sistemului/.

Peñas Defago, Maria Angelica, and Jose Morán Faúndes. 2014. "Conservative Litigation against Sexual and Reproductive Health Policies in Argentina." *Reproductive Health Matters* 22 (44): 82–90.

Penţa, Marcela, and Adriana Băban. 2013. "Dangerous Agent or Saviour? HPV Vaccine Representations on Online Discussion Forums in Romania." *International Journal of Behavioral Medicine* 21: 20–28.

Petryna, Adriana. 2003. *Life Exposed: Biological Citizens after Chernobyl.* Princeton, NJ: Princeton University Press.

Phillips, Sarah. 2002. "Half-Lives and Healthy Bodies: Discourses on 'Contaminated' Food and Healing in Post-Chernobyl Ukraine." *Food and Foodways* 10:27–53.

Pop, Cristina. n.d. "Suboptimal MMR Vaccination and Its Systemic Contingencies: A Critical Review of Romania's Measles Epidemic of 2016–2018." Unpublished manuscript.

Pop, Cristina A. 2016. "Locating Purity within Corruption Rumors: Narratives of HPV Vaccination Refusal in a Peri-Urban Community of Southern Romania." *Medical Anthropology Quarterly* 30 (4): 563–581.

Porter, Dorothy. 2011. *Health Citizenship: Essays in Social Medicine and Biomedical Politics.* Berkeley: University of California Medical Humanities Press.

Praspaliauskiene, Rima. 2016. "Enveloped Lives: Practicing Health and Care in Lithuania." *Medical Anthropology Quarterly* 30 (4): 582–598.

Preoteasa, Manuela. 2008. "Vaccinul supranumit anti-cancer. Un părinte: Dar Dvs, domnule ministru, vă asumaţi responsabilitatea?" *Hotnews.ro*, November 27. https://m.hotnews.ro/stire/5172066.

Raţ, Cristina. 2009. "Disciplining Mothers: Fertility Threats and Family Policies in Romania." In *Family Patterns and Demographic Development*, edited by N. Schleinstein, D. Sucker, A. Wenninger, and A. Wilde, 75–86. Berlin: GEISIS Leibniz Institute for Social Services.

———. 2011. "Părinţi netrebnici şi familii sănătoase. Faţa disciplinatoare a politicilor familiale." *CriticAtac*, May 31. http://www.criticatac.ro/7657/parinti-netrebnici-si-familii-sanatoase-fata-disciplinatoare-a-politicilor-familiale/.

Reeves, G. K., S.-W. Kan, T. Key, A. Tjønneland, A. Olsen, K. Overvad, P. H. Peeters, F. Clavel-Chapelon, X. Paoletti, F. Berrino, V. Krogh, D. Palli, R. Tumino, S. Panico, P. Vineis, C. A. Gonzalez, E. Ardanaz, C. Martinez, P. Amiano, J. R. Quiros, M. R. Tormo, K.-T. Khaw, A. Trichopoulou, T. Psaltopoulou, V. Kalapothaki, G. Nagel, J. Chang-Claude, H. Boeing, P. H. Lahmann, E. Wirfält, R. Kaaks, and E. Riboli. 2006. "Breast Cancer Risk in Relation to Abortion: Results from the EPIC Study." *International Journal of Cancer* 119 (7): 1741–1745.

Reich, Jennifer. 2010. "Parenting and Prevention: Views of HPV Vaccines among Parents Challenging Childhood Immunizations." In *Three Shots at Prevention: The HPV Vaccine and the Politics of Medicine's Simple Solutions*, edited by Keith Wailoo, Julie Livingston, Steve Epstein, and Robert Aronowitz, 165–181. Baltimore: Johns Hopkins University Press.

Reich, Jennifer A. 2016. "Of Natural Bodies and Antibodies: Parents' Vaccine Refusal and the Dichotomies of Natural and Artificial." *Social Science & Medicine* 157:103–110.

Renne, Elisha. 2010. *The Politics of Polio in Northern Nigeria*. Bloomington: Indiana University Press.

Rivkin-Fish, Michele. 2005. *Women's Health in Post-Soviet Russia: The Politics of Intervention*. Bloomington: Indiana University Press.

Roberts, Elizabeth F. S. 2012. *God's Laboratory: Assisted Reproduction in the Andes*. Berkeley: University of California Press.

———. 2016. "Gods, Germs, and Petri Dishes: Toward a Nonsecular Medical Anthropology." *Medical Anthropology* 35 (3): 209–219.

Roman, Denise. 2001. "Gendering Eastern Europe: Pre-Feminism, Prejudice and East-West Dialogues in Post-Communist Romania." *Women's Studies International Forum* 24 (1): 53–66.

———. 2003. *Fragmented Identities: Popular Culture, Sex, and Everyday Life in Postcommunist Romania*. Lanham, MD: Lexington Books.

Rujoiu, Valentina. 2011. "Marital Rape Law: A Comparative Approach." In *International Social Work: A Supplement of Social Work Review*, edited by Doru Buzducea, Valentina Rujoiu, Florin Lazăr, Anamaria Szabo, and Theodora Ene, 265–280. Bucharest: University of Bucharest Press.

Sahlins, Marshall. 1981. *Historical Metaphors and Mythical Realities: Structure in the Early History of the Sandwich Islands Kingdom*. Ann Arbor: University of Michigan Press.

Sam, I.-Ching, Li-Ping Wong, Sanjay Rampal, Yin-Hui Leong, Chan-Fu Pang, Yong-Ting Tai, Hwee-Ching Tee, and Maria Kahar-Bador. 2009. "Maternal Acceptance of Human Papillomavirus Vaccine in Malaysia." *Journal of Adolescent Health* 44 (6): 610–612.

Sănătate RO. 2011. "Raportul stării de sănătate România 2010." Institutul Național de Sănătate Publică. Centrul Național de Evaluare și Promovare a Stării de Sănătate (CNEPSS). https://insp.gov.ro/sites/cnepss/.

Sasson, V., and J. M. Law. 2009. *Imagining the Fetus: The Unborn in Myth, Religion, and Culture*. Oxford: Oxford University Press.

Scherb, Hagen, and Kristina Voigt. 2009. "Radiation-Induced Genetic Effects and the Chernobyl Nuclear Power Plant Accident." *Acta Paediatrica* 98:51–51.

———. 2012. "Response to W. Kramer: The Human Sex Odds at Birth after the Atmospheric Atomic Bomb Tests, after Chernobyl, and in the Vicinity of Nuclear Facilities: Comment." *Environmental Science and Pollution Research* 19 (4): 1335–1340.

Scheper-Hughes, Nancy. 1992. *Death without Weeping: The Violence of Everyday Life in Brazil*. Berkeley: University of California Press.

Scheper-Hughes, Nancy, and Margaret Lock. 1987. "The Mindful Body: A Prolegomenon to Future Work." New series, *Medical Anthropology Quarterly* 1 (1): 6–41.

Scott, James. 1985. *Weapons of the Weak: Everyday Forms of Peasant Resistance*. New Haven, CT: Yale University Press.

Șerbănescu, F., L. Morris, P. Stupp, and A. Stănescu. 1995. "The Impact of Recent Policy Changes on Fertility, Abortion, and Contraceptive Use in Romania." *Studies in Family Planning* 26 (2): 76–87.

Seymour-Smith, Charlotte. 1986. *Palgrave Dictionary of Anthropology*. London: Macmillan Press.

Simionescu, Anca, and Erika Marin. 2017. "Caesarean Birth in Romania: Safe Motherhood between Ethical, Medical and Statistical Arguments." *Maedica* 12 (1): 5–12.

Singer, Merrill. 1994. "AIDs and the Health Crisis of the U.S. Urban Poor: The Perspective of Critical Medical Anthropology." *Social Science & Medicine* 39 (7): 931–948.

Singer, Merrill, and Scott Clair. 2003. "Syndemics and Public Health: Reconceptualizing Disease in Bio-Social Context." *Medical Anthropology Quarterly* 17 (4): 423–441.

Smith, Daniel Jordan. 2008. *A Culture of Corruption: Everyday Deception and Popular Discontent in Nigeria*. Princeton, NJ: Princeton University Press.

Sobo, Elisa J. 2015. "Social Cultivation of Vaccine Refusal and Delay among Waldorf (Steiner) School Parents." *Medical Anthropology Quarterly* 29 (3): 381–399.

Stan, Lavinia, and Lucian Turcescu. 2005. "Religion, Politics and Sexuality in Romania." *Europe-Asia Studies* 57 (2): 291–310.

———. 2007. *Religion and Politics in Post-Communist Romania*. Oxford: Oxford University Press.

Stillo, Jonathan. 2010. "Magic Mountains in the Age of DOTS: Tuberculosis Sanatoria in Romania and the 'Difficult to Treat.'" Paper presented at the American Anthropological Association Annual Meeting, New Orleans.

———. 2011. "The Romanian Tuberculosis Epidemic as a Symbol of Public Health." In *Romania under Basescu: Aspirations, Achievements and Frustrations during His First Presidential Term*, edited by Ronald King and Paul Sum, 273–292. Lanham, MD: Lexington Books.

Stoicescu, M., G. Bungau, D. Țit, G. Mutiu, A. Purza, V. Iovan, and O. Pop. 2017. "Carcinogenic Uterine Risk of Repeated Abortions: Hormone Receptors Tumoral Expression." *Romanian Journal of Morphology & Embryology* 58 (4): 1429–1434.

Stone, Linda. 2006. *Kinship and Gender: An Introduction*. Boulder, CO: Westview Press.

Swaddiwudhipong, W., C. Chaovakiratipong, P. Nguntra, P. Mahasakpan, Y. Tatip, and C. Boonmak. 1999. "A Mobile Unit: An Effective Service for Cervical Cancer Screening among Rural Thai Women." *International Journal of Epidemiology* 28 (1): 35–39.

Temkina, Anna, and Michele Rivkin-Fish. 2020. "Creating Health Care Consumers: The Negotiation of Un/Official Payments, Power and Trust in Russian Maternity Care." *Social Theory & Health* 18:340–357.

Tismăneanu, Vladimir. 2003. *Stalinism for All Seasons: A Political History of Romanian Communism*. Berkeley: University of California Press.

Todorova, Irina, Adriana Băban, Dina Balabanova, Yulia Panayotova, and Janet Bradley. 2006. "Providers' Constructions of the Role of Women in Cervical Cancer Screening in Bulgaria and Romania." *Social Science & Medicine* 63:776–787.

Todorova, Maria. 1997. *Imagining the Balkans*. New York: Oxford University Press.

Towghi, Fouzieyha. 2010. "Circulation of Therapeutic Norms against Cervical Cancer and Globalization of Market for HPV Vaccines." Paper presented at the American Anthropological Association Annual Meeting, New Orleans.

———. 2013. "The Biopolitics of Reproductive Technologies beyond the Clinic: Localizing HPV Vaccines in India." *Medical Anthropology* 32 (4): 325–342.

Trnka, Susanna. 2007. "Languages of Labor: Negotiating the 'Real' and the Relational in Indo-Fijian Women's Expressions of Physical Pain." *Medical Anthropology Quarterly* 21 (4): 388–408.

Tudorică, Andreea. 2017. "România, campioană la cezariene." *Cotidianul.ro*, September 3. https://www.cotidianul.ro/romania-campioana-la-cezariene/.

Van der Kolk, Bessel. 2014. *The Body Keeps the Score: Brain, Mind, and Body in the Healing of Trauma*. New York: Penguin Books.

Van Maanen, John. 2011. *Tales of the Field: On Writing Ethnography.* 2nd ed. Chicago: University of Chicago Press.

Varley, Emma, and Saiba Varma. 2018. "Spectral Ties: Hospital Hauntings across the Line of Control." *Medical Anthropology* 37 (8): 630–644.

Vassilev, Dimiter. 1999. "Bulgaria." In *From Abortion to Contraception: A Resource to Public Policies and Reproductive Behavior in Central and Eastern Europe from 1917 to the Present,* edited by Henry P. David, 69–90. Westport, CT: Greenwood.

Verdery, Katherine. 1996. *What Was Socialism, and What Comes Next?* Princeton, NJ: Princeton University Press.

Vlădescu, C., G. Scîntee, V. Olsavszky, S. Allin, and P. Mladovsky. 2008. "Romania: Health System Review." *Health Systems in Transition* 10 (3): 1–172.

Vlădescu, Cristian. 2009. "Migration of Nurses: The Case of Romania." *Management in Health* 13 (4): 12–16.

Vlaston, Ștefan. 2011. "Este "privatizarea" sistemelor de sănătate și educație o soluție?" *Contributors.ro,* September 13. https://www.contributors.ro/este-privatizarea-sistemelor-de-sanatate-si-educatie-o-solutie/.

Voland, Eckhart, and Jan Beise. 2005. "The Husband's Mother Is the Devil in the House: Data on the Impact of the Mother-in-Law on Stillbirth Mortality in Historical Krummhorn (1750–1874) and Some Thoughts on the Evolution of Postgenerative Female Life." In *Grandmotherhood: The Evolutionary Significance of the Second Half of Female Life,* edited by Eckart Voland, Anthanasios Chasiotis, and Wulf Schiefenhovel, 239–255. New Brunswick, NJ: Rutgers University Press.

Wailoo, Keith, Julie Livingston, Steve Epstein, and Robert Aronowitz, eds. 2010. *Three Shots at Prevention: The HPV Vaccine and the Politics of Medicine's Simple Solutions.* Baltimore: Johns Hopkins University Press.

Webster, Joseph. 2013. *The Anthropology of Protestantism: Faith and Crisis among Scottish Fishermen.* New York: Palgrave Macmillan.

Weiner, Noga. 2009. "The Intensive Medical Care of Sick, Impaired, and Preterm Newborns in Israel and the Production of Vulnerable Neonatal Subjectivities." *Medical Anthropology Quarterly* 23 (3): 320–341.

Wentzell, Emily. 2013. "Aging Respectably by Rejecting Medicalization: Mexican Men's Reasons for Not Using Erectile Dysfunction Drugs." *Medical Anthropology Quarterly* 27 (1): 3–22.

White, Luise. 1995. "Tsetse Visions: Narratives of Blood and Bugs in Colonial Northern Rhodesia, 1931–9." *Journal of African History* 36 (2): 219–245.

———. 2000. *Speaking with Vampires: Rumor and History in Colonial Africa.* Berkeley: University of California Press.

Whitmarsh, Ian, and Elizabeth Roberts. 2016. "Nonsecular Medical Anthropology." *Medical Anthropology* 35 (3): 203–208.

Williams, Raymond, and Michael Orrom. 1954. *Preface to Film.* London: Film Drama Limited.

Wilson, Caroline. 2010. "'Eating, eating is always there': Food, consumerism and cardiovascular disease. Some evidence from Kerala, South India." *Anthropology and Medicine* 17 (3): 261–275.

Wood, Katherine, Rachel Jewkes, and Naeemah Abrahams. 1997. "Cleaning the Womb: Constructions of Cervical Screening and Womb Cancer among Rural Black Women in South Africa." *Social Science & Medicine* 45 (2): 283–294.

Zafiu, Rodica. 2010. *101 Cuvinte Argotice.* București: Humanitas.

Zerilli, Filippo M. 2005. "Corruption, Property Restitution and Romanianness" In *Corruption: Anthropological Perspectives,* edited by Dieter Haller and Chris Shore, 83–102. London: Pluto Press.

INDEX

Page numbers in *italic* refer to illustrations or tables.

vaccines, 112–115. *See also* HPV (human
papillomavirus)
Vasilica (study participant), 129–130, 149
Venezuela, 6, 7
Veronica (study participant), 157–158
Veturia (study participant), 32, 77, 83
virginity and HPV vaccine, 164–166

Warren, Narelle, 8
water and sewers, 15

White, Luise, 160
WHO European Region, 2
women, triple burden of, 23, 37, 50
women's rights, 26–27, 26
"working comrades," 26

Xenia (subject of urban legend), 9, 13,
158–159

Zerilli, Filippo M., 160

ABOUT THE AUTHOR

CRISTINA A. POP is an assistant professor of medical anthropology at Creighton University in Omaha, Nebraska. She has published her research in *Medical Anthropology Quarterly*, *Medical Anthropology*, *Journal of Religion and Health*, and *Culture, Health and Sexuality*.